mix 'n match
meals in
minutes

for people with diabetes

Linda Gassenheimer

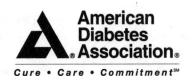

American
Diabetes
Association®

Cure • Care • Commitment℠

Director, Book Publishing, John Fedor; *Associate Director, Consumer Books,* Sherrye Landrum; *Editor,* Laurie Guffey; *Production Manager,* Peggy M. Rote; *Composition,* Circle Graphics; *Cover Design,* Koncept, Inc.; *Cover Photography,* Paul Rubiera; *Food Stylist,* Ellen Stern; *Nutritional Analysis,* Nutritional Computing Concepts, Inc.; *Printer,* Port City Press, Inc.

Printed in the United States of America
1 3 5 7 9 10 8 6 4 2

The suggestions and information contained in this publication are generally consistent with the *Clinical Practice Recommendations* and other policies of the American Diabetes Association, but they do not represent the policy or position of the Association or any of its boards or committees. Reasonable steps have been taken to ensure the accuracy of the information presented. However, the American Diabetes Association cannot ensure the safety or efficacy of any product or service described in this publication. Individuals are advised to consult a physician or other appropriate health care professional before undertaking any diet or exercise program or taking any medication referred to in this publication. Professionals must use and apply their own professional judgment, experience, and training and should not rely solely on the information contained in this publication before prescribing any diet, exercise, or medication. The American Diabetes Association—its officers, directors, employees, volunteers, and members—assumes no responsibility or liability for personal or other injury, loss, or damage that may result from the suggestions or information in this publication.

⊚ The paper in this publication meets the requirements of the ANSI Standard Z39.48-1992 (permanence of paper).

ADA titles may be purchased for business or promotional use or for special sales. To purchase this book in large quantities, or for custom editions of this book with your logo, contact Lee Romano Sequeira, Special Sales & Promotions, at the address below, or at LRomano@diabetes.org or 703-299-2046.

American Diabetes Association
1701 North Beauregard Street
Alexandria, Virginia 22311

Library of Congress Cataloging-in-Publication Data

Gassenheimer, Linda.
    Mix 'n match meals in minutes for people with diabetes / Linda Gassenheimer.
       p. cm.
    Includes index.
    ISBN 1-58040-171-6 (pbk. : alk. paper)
      1. Diabetes—Diet therapy—Recipes. I. Title: Mix and match meals in minutes for people with diabetes. II. American Diabetes Association. III. Title.

RC662.G37 2003
641.5'6314—dc21

2002043719

On the cover: *Neopolitan Pizza,* page 76; *Claudine's Tilapia* with *Saffron Broccoli and Potatoes,* page 156; *Cider Pork* with *Autumn Squash,* page 138; and back cover, *Ginger-Minted Chicken* with *Lemon and Carrot Barley* and *Honey Pecan Peaches,* page 108.

To my husband, Harold,
for his encouragement, help, and support.

contents

acknowledgments

Many thanks go to my husband, Harold. He has patiently edited every word and provided the analysis that helped structure these recipes.

Affectionate thank yous go to those whose guidance and support helped me to create this book:

My assistant, Jackie Murrill, who has been a wonderful help, spending hours with me testing recipes—and always with a smile.

Lynne Stein, Senior Program Manager for the American Diabetes Association in Miami, who encouraged me to write this book.

Maria Elena Torres, ARNP, MSN, CDE, and Marayxa Suarez, RD, LD, MS, CDE, are educators whose infectious enthusiasm and guidance were an invaluable aide to understanding the issues faced by those with diabetes.

My editors, Sherrye Landrum and Laurie Guffey, whose support and friendship have made working on this book a delight.

My family, who always encourage my projects. My son James, his wife Patty, and their sons, Zachary and Jacob, all came for dinner with a smile. My son John, his wife Jill, and their children, Jeffrey and Joanna, and my son Charles and his wife Lori all cheered me on. My sister Roberta and brother-in-law Robert helped to edit my thoughts and words.

Kathy Martin, my editor at the *Miami Herald*, who has enthusiastically encouraged my work.

Joseph Cooper and the management and staff at WLRN 91.3 FM, public radio for South Florida, for their friendship and help.

And all of you who use this book and prepare these meals: I hope you enjoy them as much as I've enjoyed creating these recipes!

introduction

Three years ago my sister called me, saying she had just come from the doctor's office with the news that she had type 2 diabetes. She bombarded me with questions: "What do I eat? Where do I start? What's on the list and what's off the list? How can I fit this style of eating into my busy life?"

Just last month one of my friends called me. Her husband had just come home with the same news. Her questions were identical to my sister's. A dietitian at the hospital had given her some guidelines, but she needed to translate them into simple, quick meals. "What should I buy at the supermarket? How can I make tasty meals that will satisfy my husband?"

What my sister and friend—and perhaps you, too—need is a blueprint of what to have on hand, what to buy, and how to put ingredients together for quick, healthy, and delicious meals. I've provided a blueprint that is flexible, so you can mix and match your favorite meals, and structured, so you don't have to spend a lot of time planning what to serve. Diabetes doesn't mean broiled chicken every night—I've provided a wide variety of meals with many ethnic flavors. My main goal is for you to enjoy the recipes and know that you can still have delicious and exciting meals.

These are easy-to-follow recipes. From years of training, I've learned to use classic techniques and familiar combinations to produce delicious results while cutting the cooking time. Some recipes take as little as 15 minutes to make. Others take longer, but are worth the time when you have it. When you're in a hurry, just repeat one of the quick recipes you enjoy and save the longer ones for the weekend or another weekday meal.

My method will save you time in the kitchen and at the grocery store. I've provided complete shopping lists, helpful hints, and a countdown section so you know exactly how to time your cooking so the whole meal is done at once. I developed these techniques after many years of juggling my family and career (founding and running a cooking school, guiding a gourmet supermarket, writing food columns for newspapers and magazines, and hosting a radio talk show), while still wanting to eat well!

Shopping List

I've based my list based on how you buy food in the supermarket.

▌ Quick shopping is as important as quick cooking. You won't have to think about how many mushrooms to buy. I've given you the amount.

▌ I list the ingredients by supermarket departments to help you navigate the aisles with ease.

▌ Shopping lists will save you both time and money, since you buy only what you need.

▌ My staples list helps you organize your cabinets so they are not filled with unused items. To help you begin, I've included a list of all the staples I call for in the recipes (see page xii). You probably already have many of these ingredients on hand and only need to buy a few fresh items.

Helpful Hints and Countdowns

Each meal contains tips on shopping, cooking, and substitutions, and a count-down so you can get the whole meal on the table at the same time.

▌ You can hit the kitchen on the run without having to plan or think about each step.

▌ My prep times begin when I turn on the light in the kitchen and end when I bring the plates to the table.

▌ Helpful hints tell you what to buy, how to buy it, and what you can substitute. They include tips on the best preparation and quick-cooking techniques and how to save cleanup time.

Flexible Recipes

You can dress up these recipes for company, or dress them down to suit your budget.

▌ You can use the best sirloin, filet, or strip steak, or more economical cuts like flank and skirt steaks.

▌ You can use gourmet ingredients like infused olive oil or aged balsamic vinegar, or achieve delicious results with products you have on hand.

▌ When you choose a fish recipe, you can buy the freshest-looking fish in the market rather than the fish called for in the recipe.

| My flexible recipes let you choose whatever is in season, on sale, looks most appealing, or fits your mood.

As you go through the recipes, keep a few things in mind. All the recipes serve two people. The nutrient analyses for the recipes were calculated using Paul Newman's salad dressings, whole-wheat bread, and All-Bran Bran Buds cereal. You can use any type of oil and vinegar dressing, whole-wheat bread, and bran cereal you like, but the nutrient values will vary from those given. "Salt and pepper to taste" are NOT included in the analyses. Finally, a few of these recipes are high in sodium. If you need to watch your sodium levels, check those values carefully. These meals (any one breakfast, lunch, and dinner together) average about 1350 calories and 165 grams of carbohydrate a day.

More Helpful Hints

Below are some general tips to help you eat well and cook like an expert!

Buying Tips

| Buy good-quality Parmesan cheese and ask the market to grate it for you or chop it in the food processor. Freeze extra for quick use. You can spoon out what you need and leave the rest frozen.
| Fresh fish should be firm to the touch and have a sweet smell. If it is whole, in addition to firm flesh, the eyes should be clear and the gills red.
| Buy shelled shrimp or ask for the shrimp to be shelled when you buy it. Many supermarkets will do this for a small fee. I find the slightly higher cost is worth the time saved.
| Buy tomato paste in a tube. You can use a small amount and the rest of the tube can be stored in the refrigerator until needed again.
| If you use dried herbs, make sure they are no more than six months old. They lose their flavor if kept too long.
| Brown rice takes about 45 minutes to cook, but there are several brands of quick-cooking brown rice available. Their cooking time ranges from 10 minutes to 30 minutes. I find the 30-minute rice has more flavor, but you can use any quick-cooking rice and follow package cooking directions.
| I call for a small amount of wine, liquor, or liqueur in some recipes. If you don't have any on hand, you can buy small bottles or splits at most liquor stores.

Preparation Tips

▌ To quickly chop fresh herbs, wash and dry them and snip the leaves with scissors.

▌ To quickly peel ginger, scrape the skin away with the edge of a spoon.

▌ To quickly chop ginger, place small, peeled pieces in a garlic press with large holes. Press over a bowl to catch the juices.

Cooking Methods

Stir-Frying

▌ Make sure your wok is very hot before you add the ingredients.

▌ The secret to crisp, not steamed, stir-frying is to let the ingredients sit for about a minute when you add them to the hot wok before you toss them. This allows the wok to regain its heat after the cold ingredients have been added.

▌ For easy stir-frying, place all of the prepared ingredients on a cutting board or plate in order of use. You won't have to look at the recipe once you start to cook.

Cooking Fish

▌ Count 10 minutes cooking time for each inch of thickness. To check for doneness, stick the point of a knife into the flesh. If the flesh is opaque, it is ready.

▌ Remember the fish will continue to cook after it has been removed from the heat. Do not overcook, or the fish will be dry and tasteless.

Cooking Pasta

▌ Always use a very large pot. The pasta should be able to roll freely as it cooks.

▌ Make sure the water is at a rolling boil before you add the pasta.

▌ Add the pasta at one time and stir once.

Cooking Staples

Keep these foods on hand in your pantry or fridge, and you'll only have to pick up a few items at the supermarket to complete your meals.

Dairy

Eggs

Parmesan cheese

Butter

Fat-free milk

Grocery

Grains

Quick-cooking brown rice   Long-grain white rice

Spices

Salt
Black peppercorns   Chili powder
Ground cinnamon   Ground cumin seed

Breads and Cereals

Plain bread crumbs   Oatmeal
Whole-wheat bread   Bran cereal

Condiments

Reduced-fat mayonnaise   Hot pepper sauce
Dijon mustard   Worcestershire sauce
Ketchup   Lite soy sauce

Oils, Vinegars, and Dressings

Canola oil   White vinegar
Sesame oil   Cider vinegar
Olive oil   Paul Newman's Oil and
Vegetable oil cooking spray   Vinegar Salad Dressing
Olive oil cooking spray   Paul Newman's Oil and
Balsamic vinegar   Balsamic Vinegar Salad Dressing

Miscellaneous

Sugar substitute   Instant decaffeinated coffee
Cornstarch   Vanilla extract
Raisins   Orange juice
Fat-free reduced-sodium chicken broth   Extra-dry vermouth

Produce

Garlic   Red onion   Onion   Celery
Lemon   Carrots   Apples

A Month of Meals at a Glance

All of the breakfasts, lunches, and dinners can be mixed and matched according to your preference. Below is just one example of a tasty month of meals. I have organized them into a meal-at-a-glance chart, with some easy and quick meals midweek and those that take a little more time on the weekends. They are arranged to give variety throughout the day and over the days of the week.

Week 1	Sunday	Monday	Tuesday	Wednesday	Thursday	Friday	Saturday
Breakfast	Nutty Cinnamon French Toast, p. 30	Fluffy Scramble, p. 2	Spicy Grilled Cheese and Tomato Sandwich, p. 22	Breakfast Egg Sandwich, p. 20	Blueberry Smoothie, p. 24	Toasted Turkey Breakfast Sandwich, p. 28	Parmesan Frittata, p. 6
Lunch	Shrimp and Black-Eyed Pea Salad, p. 36	Italian Hero Sandwich, p. 58	Grilled Turkey Sausage, p. 60	Shrimp Roll, p. 62	Quick Turkey Wrap, p. 64	Tuscan Bean and Tuna Salad, p. 38	Antipasto Platter, p. 40
Dinner	Honey Mustard Beef Kabobs, p. 117	Baked Shrimp, p. 144	Chinese Steamed Fish, p. 147	Middle Eastern Meatballs, p. 114	Chinese Pepper Steak, p. 120	Wok-Flashed Shrimp, p. 150	Korean Grilled Beef, p. 123

Week 2	Sunday	Monday	Tuesday	Wednesday	Thursday	Friday	Saturday
Breakfast	Basque Red Pepper Frittata, p. 8	Spicy Grilled Cheese and Tomato Sandwich, p. 22	Microwave Ham-Scrambled Eggs, p. 4	Toasted Turkey Breakfast Sandwich, p. 28	Spinach and Mushroom Omelet, p. 16	Blueberry Smoothie, p. 24	Norwegian Bagel Breakfast, p. 26
Lunch	Horace's Chickpea Soup, p. 82	Shrimp Caesar Salad, p. 42	Chicken Avocado Wrap, p. 66	Ham, Swiss, Apple, and Spinach Salad, p. 35	Mediterranean Egg Salad Sandwich, p. 68	Sausage and Tortellini Soup, p. 84	Smoked Fish Salad, p. 44
Dinner	Stuffed Veal Rolls, p. 129	Chinese Chicken with Cashew Nuts, p. 93	Italian Fish Soup, p. 153	Claudine's Tilapia, p. 156	Picadillo, p. 126	Crisp Thai Snapper, p. 159	Veal Gorgonzola, p. 132

A Month of Meals at a Glance (*Continued*)

Week 3	Sunday	Monday	Tuesday	Wednesday	Thursday	Friday	Saturday
Breakfast	Smoked Salmon Omelet, p. 18	Fluffy Scramble, p. 2	Norwegian Bagel Breakfast, p. 26	Spicy Grilled Cheese and Tomato Sandwich, p. 22	Microwave Ham-Scrambled Eggs, p. 4	Toasted Turkey Breakfast Sandwich, p. 28	Tomato, Onion, and Basil Frittata, p. 10
Lunch	Steak and Portobello Mushroom Sandwich, p. 70	Turkey and Vegetable Soup, p. 86	Smoked Turkey Waldorf Salad, p. 46	Italian Peasant Salad, p. 48	Crunchy Coleslaw and Turkey Sandwich, p. 72	Roast Beef Sandwich, p. 74	Pasta and Bean Soup, p. 88
Dinner	Mojo Roasted Pork, p. 135	Southwestern Chicken, p. 96	Hungarian Goulash, p. 99	Chicken Cacciatore, p. 102	Seafood Kabobs, p. 162	Cider Pork, p. 138	Sautéed Scallops, p. 165

Week 4	Sunday	Monday	Tuesday	Wednesday	Thursday	Friday	Saturday
Breakfast	Spinach and Mushroom Omelet, p. 16	Toasted Turkey Breakfast Sandwich, p. 28	Gorgonzola Omelet, p. 14	Spicy Grilled Cheese and Tomato Sandwich, p. 22	Blueberry Smoothie, p. 24	Swiss Omelet, p. 12	Nutty Cinnamon French Toast, p. 30
Lunch	Neapolitan Pizza, p. 76	Toasted Almond Chicken Salad, p. 50	Turkey and Goat Cheese Enchiladas, p. 78	Salsa Beef Salad, p. 52	Chef's Salad, p. 54	Greek Tuna Salad Pita Pocket, p. 80	Tangy Chicken and Pear Salad, p. 56
Dinner	Shrimp Creole, p. 168	Mediterranean Meat Loaf, p. 105	Herb-Crusted Mahi-Mahi, p. 171	Key West Shrimp, p. 174	Ginger-Minted Chicken, p. 108	Turkey Chili, p. 111	Italian Roast Pork, p. 141

breakfast

fluffy scramble

Fluffy Scramble
Oatmeal

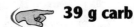 **39 g carb**

The secret to these light, fluffy scrambled eggs is whisking soft tofu into the eggs. A hint of cayenne pepper and Dijon mustard add a little bite.

HELPFUL HINT

❚ Soft tofu can be found in the refrigerated case of the produce section of most supermarkets.

COUNTDOWN

❚ Make oatmeal
❚ Toast bread
❚ Make eggs

Fluffy Scramble

Prep time: **10 minutes**
Serves 2/Serving size: **1/2 recipe**

2 slices whole-wheat bread
Olive oil cooking spray
2 whole eggs
2 egg whites
2 oz soft tofu (1/4 cup)
Pinch cayenne pepper
1 Tbsp Dijon mustard
Salt and freshly ground black pepper to taste

Exchanges
1 Starch
2 Lean Meat

Calories 185
  Calories from Fat . . 67
Total Fat. . . . . 7 g
  Saturated Fat. . . . . . 2 g
Cholesterol. . . . . . 213 mg
Sodium. . . . . 446 mg
Carbohydrate. . . . . 15 g
  Dietary Fiber . . . . . . 2 g
  Sugars. . . . . 4 g
Protein. . . . . 15 g

1. Toast bread. Spray one side of each slice with cooking spray and place on 2 plates.
2. Whisk whole eggs, egg whites, tofu, cayenne pepper, and mustard in a blender, food processor, or bowl. Add salt and pepper.
3. Heat a nonstick skillet over medium-high heat. Spray with cooking spray.
4. Add egg mixture and scramble eggs 1 minute. Remove and serve on toasted bread.

Oatmeal

Preparation time: **5 minutes**
Serves 2/Serving size: **1/2 cup**

2/3 cup oatmeal
1 cup water
1 cup fat-free milk

1. Place oatmeal in a microwave-safe bowl and add water.
2. Microwave on high 3 minutes.
3. Place in 2 bowls and serve with milk.

Exchanges
1 Starch
1/2 Fat-Free Milk

Calories 147
Calories from Fat . . 17
Total Fat. . . . . 2 g
Saturated Fat. . . . . . 0 g
Cholesterol. . . . . . . 2 mg
Sodium. . . . . 64 mg
Carbohydrate. . . . . 24 g
Dietary Fiber . . . . . . 3 g
Sugars. . . . . 6 g
Protein. . . . . 9 g

SHOPPING LIST

STAPLES

Produce
1 small package soft tofu

Eggs (4 needed)
Dijon mustard
Cayenne pepper
Oatmeal
Fat-free milk

Whole-wheat bread
Olive oil cooking spray
Salt
Black peppercorns

ham-scrambled eggs

**Microwave Ham-Scrambled Eggs
Oatmeal**

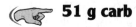 **51 g carb**

Scrambled eggs and ham in less than 3 minutes and no pan to wash! It's easy with this recipe.

HELPFUL HINT

▌ Microwave timing may vary with different microwave ovens, so change your timing accordingly.

COUNTDOWN

▌ Make oatmeal
▌ Make eggs
▌ Toast bread

Microwave Ham-Scrambled Eggs

Preparation time: **10 minutes**
Serves 2/serving size: **1/2 recipe**

2 eggs
4 egg whites
2 oz lean ham torn into bite-sized pieces (1/2 cup)
 Salt and freshly ground black pepper to taste
4 slices whole-wheat bread

Exchanges
2 Starch
2 Lean Meat
1/2 Fat

Calories 291
 Calories from Fat . . 81
Total Fat. . . . . 9 g
 Saturated Fat. . . . . . 2 g
Cholesterol. . . . . . 229 mg
Sodium. . . . . 845 mg
Carbohydrate. . . . . 27 g
 Dietary Fiber . . . . . . 4 g
 Sugars. . . . . 4 g
Protein. . . . . 26 g

1. Mix 1 whole egg, 2 egg whites, and half the ham pieces together in a microwave-safe bowl; repeat with remaining ingredients in a second bowl.
2. Add salt and pepper to both.
3. Microwave first bowl on high for 1 minute. Stir and return for 30 seconds; repeat with second serving.
4. Toast bread and serve with ham and eggs.

Oatmeal

Preparation time: **5 minutes**
Serves 2/Serving size: **1/2 cup**

2/3 cup oatmeal
 1 cup water
 1 cup fat-free milk

1. Place oatmeal in a microwave-safe bowl and add water.
2. Microwave on high 3 minutes.
3. Place in 2 bowls and serve with milk.

Exchanges
1 Starch
1/2 Fat-Free Milk

Calories 147
 Calories from Fat . . 17
Total Fat. . . . . 2 g
 Saturated Fat. . . . . . 0 g
Cholesterol. . . . . . . 2 mg
Sodium. . . . . 64 mg
Carbohydrate. . . . . 24 g
 Dietary Fiber . . . . . . 3 g
 Sugars. . . . . 6 g
Protein. . . . . 9 g

SHOPPING LIST

Deli
1 small package lean
 ham

STAPLES

Eggs (6 needed)
Whole-wheat bread
Oatmeal
Fat-free milk
Salt
Black peppercorns

parmesan frittata

Parmesan Frittata
Oatmeal

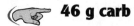 **46 g carb**

Plump, flavorful frittatas make a nice breakfast change. They take a little longer to make than scrambled eggs or omelets. Make them on the weekend, or make them the night before and heat them in the microwave the next morning.

Frittatas are different from omelets. A frittata is cooked very slowly over low heat, making it firm and set, while an omelet is cooked fast over high heat, making it more creamy and runny. A frittata needs to be cooked on both sides. Some people flip it in the pan, but a much easier way is to place it under the broiler for half a minute. Here is a basic cheese frittata recipe followed by several variations.

HELPFUL HINT

▌ Buy good-quality Parmesan cheese and ask the market to grate it for you or chop it in the food processor. Freeze extra for quick use. You can spoon out the quantity you need and leave the rest frozen.

COUNTDOWN

▌ Preheat broiler
▌ Make toast
▌ Make frittata
▌ Make oatmeal

Parmesan Frittata

Preparation time: **20 minutes**
Serves 2/Serving size: **1/2 recipe**

2 slices whole-wheat bread
   Olive oil cooking spray
2 whole eggs
4 egg whites
1/4 cup grated Parmesan cheese
1 cup frozen chopped onion
   Salt and freshly ground black pepper to taste

1. Preheat broiler. Toast bread and spray one side of each slice with cooking spray.
2. Mix whole eggs, egg whites, Parmesan cheese, and onion together. Add salt and pepper.
3. Heat a 9- or 10-inch nonstick oven-safe skillet over medium-low heat and spray with cooking spray. Add egg mixture and turn the heat down to low.
4. Cook eggs without browning the bottom for 10 minutes. The eggs will be set, but the top will be a little runny.
5. Place pan under the broiler for 30 seconds to 1 minute until the top is set, but not brown. Remove and cut in half. Slide halves onto 2 plates and serve with toast.

Exchanges

| 1 Starch | 2 Lean Meat |
| 1 Vegetable | 1 Fat |

Calories 258
 Calories from Fat . . 89
Total Fat . . . . 10 g
 Saturated Fat . . . . . . 4 g
Cholesterol . . . . . . 223 mg
Sodium . . . . 413 mg
Carbohydrate . . . . . 22 g
 Dietary Fiber . . . . . . 3 g
 Sugars . . . . 8 g
Protein . . . . 21 g

EGGS

Oatmeal

Preparation time: **5 minutes**
Serves 2/Serving size: **1/2 cup**

2/3 cup oatmeal
 1 cup water
 1 cup fat-free milk

1. Place oatmeal in a microwave-safe bowl and add water.
2. Microwave on high 3 minutes.
3. Place in 2 bowls and serve with milk.

Exchanges

| 1 Starch | 1/2 Fat-Free Milk |

Calories 147
 Calories from Fat . . 17
Total Fat . . . . 2 g
 Saturated Fat . . . . . . 0 g
Cholesterol . . . . 2 mg
Sodium . . . . 64 mg
Carbohydrate . . . . . 24 g
 Dietary Fiber . . . . . . 3 g
 Sugars . . . . 6 g
Protein . . . . 9 g

SHOPPING LIST

Dairy
1 small piece Parmesan cheese

Grocery
Frozen chopped onion

STAPLES

Eggs (6 needed)
Whole-wheat bread
Olive oil cooking spray
Oatmeal

Fat-free milk
Salt
Black peppercorns

basque frittata

Basque Red Pepper Frittata
Oatmeal

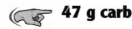 **47 g carb**

COUNTDOWN

▌ Microwave vegetables
▌ Make toast
▌ Preheat broiler
▌ Make frittata
▌ Make oatmeal

Basque Red Pepper Frittata

Preparation time: **20 minutes**
Serves 2/Serving size: **1/2 recipe**

1 cup thinly sliced red bell peppers
2 plum tomatoes, thinly sliced
2 medium cloves garlic, crushed
2 slices whole-wheat bread
  Olive oil cooking spray
2 whole eggs
4 egg whites
  Salt and freshly ground black pepper to taste

1. Place red peppers, tomatoes and garlic in a microwave-safe bowl. Microwave on high 5 minutes.
2. Meanwhile, toast bread and spray one side of each slice with olive oil cooking spray. Set aside.
3. Preheat broiler. Mix whole eggs and egg whites together. Add vegetables, salt, and pepper.

Exchanges
1 Starch
2 Lean Meat
1 Vegetable

Calories	215
Calories from Fat . .	59
Total Fat.	7 g
Saturated Fat.	2 g
Cholesterol.	213 mg
Sodium.	331 mg
Carbohydrate.	23 g
Dietary Fiber	4 g
Sugars.	7 g
Protein.	17 g

4. Heat a 9- or 10-inch nonstick skillet over medium-low heat and spray with olive oil cooking spray. Add egg mixture and turn the heat down to low.
5. Cook without browning the bottom 10 minutes. The eggs will be set, but the top will be a little runny.
6. Place pan under the broiler for 30 seconds to 1 minute until the top is set, but not brown. Remove and cut in half. Slide halves onto 2 plates and serve with toast.

Oatmeal

Preparation time: **5 minutes**
Serves 2/Serving size: **1/2 cup**

2/3 cup oatmeal
1 cup water
1 cup fat-free milk

1. Place oatmeal in a microwave-safe bowl and add water.
2. Microwave on high 3 minutes.
3. Place in 2 bowls and serve with milk.

Exchanges
1 Starch
1/2 Fat-Free Milk

Calories 147
   Calories from Fat . . 17
Total Fat. . . . . 2 g
   Saturated Fat. . . . . . 0 g
Cholesterol. . . . . . . 2 mg
Sodium. . . . . 64 mg
Carbohydrate. . . . . 24 g
   Dietary Fiber . . . . . . 3 g
   Sugars. . . . . 6 g
Protein. . . . . 9 g

SHOPPING LIST

Produce
1 large red bell pepper
2 plum tomatoes

STAPLES

Eggs (6 needed)
Garlic
Whole-wheat bread
Oatmeal

Fat-free milk
Olive oil cooking spray
Salt
Black peppercorns

tomato frittata

Tomato, Onion, and Basil Frittata
Oatmeal

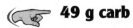 **49 g carb**

COUNTDOWN

▌ Microwave vegetables
▌ Make toast
▌ Preheat broiler
▌ Make frittata
▌ Make oatmeal

Tomato, Onion, and Basil Frittata

Preparation time: **20 minutes**
Serves 2/Serving size: **1/2 recipe**

1 cup thinly sliced red onion
1 cup canned whole tomatoes, drained
1 cup fresh basil leaves, torn into bite-sized pieces
2 slices whole-wheat bread
   Olive oil cooking spray
2 whole eggs
4 egg whites
   Salt and freshly ground black pepper to taste

1. Place onion and tomatoes in a microwave-safe
   bowl. Break up the tomatoes with the edge
   of a spoon. Microwave on high 5 minutes.
   Remove from microwave and add basil.
2. Toast bread and spray one side of each slice
   with cooking spray.
3. Preheat broiler. Mix whole eggs and egg whites
   together. Add onion, tomatoes, salt, and pepper.
4. Heat a 9- or 10-inch nonstick skillet over
   medium-low heat. Add egg mixture and turn
   the heat down to low.

Exchanges
1 Starch
2 Lean Meat
1 Vegetable

Calories 231
   Calories from Fat . . 58
Total Fat. . . . . 6 g
   Saturated Fat . . . . . . 2 g
Cholesterol. . . . . . 213 mg
Sodium. . . . . 500 mg
Carbohydrate. . . . . 25 g
   Dietary Fiber . . . . . . 5 g
   Sugars. . . . . 9 g
Protein. . . . . 19 g

5. Cook without browning the bottom 10 minutes. The eggs will be set, but the top will be a little runny.
6. Place pan under the broiler for 30 seconds to 1 minute until the top is set, but not brown. Remove and cut in half. Slide halves onto 2 plates and serve with toast.

Oatmeal

Preparation time: **5 minutes**
Serves 2/Serving size: **1/2 cup**

2/3 cup oatmeal
1 cup water
1 cup fat-free milk

1. Place oatmeal in a microwave-safe bowl and add water.
2. Microwave on high 3 minutes.
3. Place in 2 bowls and serve with milk.

Exchanges
1 Starch
1/2 Fat-Free Milk

Calories 147
  Calories from Fat . . 17
Total Fat . . . . 2 g
  Saturated Fat . . . . . . 0 g
Cholesterol . . . . 2 mg
Sodium . . . . 64 mg
Carbohydrate . . . . . 24 g
  Dietary Fiber . . . . . . 3 g
  Sugars . . . . 6 g
Protein . . . . 9 g

SHOPPING LIST

Produce
1 red onion
1 small bunch basil

Grocery
1 small can whole tomatoes

STAPLES

Eggs (6 needed)
Whole-wheat bread
Olive oil cooking spray
Oatmeal
Fat-free milk
Salt
Black peppercorns

swiss omelet

Swiss Omelet
Bran Cereal

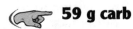 **59 g carb**

A perfect omelet is golden on the top with a delicate creamy center. The secret is to cook it over medium-high heat for only a couple of minutes. Here is a basic cheese omelet recipe followed by several variations.

HELPFUL HINT

▌ Slightly shake the pan while the omelet cooks to help set all of the egg. This also helps make the omelet a little thicker.

COUNTDOWN

▌ Toast bread
▌ Make omelet
▌ Assemble cereal

Swiss Omelet

Preparation time: **10 minutes**
Serves 2/serving size: **1/2 recipe**

2 slices rye bread
Olive oil cooking spray
2 cups egg substitute
Pinch cayenne
Salt and freshly ground black pepper to taste
2 oz reduced-fat Swiss cheese torn into bite-sized pieces
(1/2 cup)

1. Toast bread and spray one side of each slice with olive oil cooking spray. Set aside.
2. Pour egg substitute into a bowl and stir in cayenne pepper, salt, and pepper.
3. Heat a 9- or 10-inch nonstick skillet over medium-high heat and spray with cooking spray. Pour in egg mixture. Let eggs set for about 30 seconds. Tip the pan and lightly move the eggs so that they all set. Cook 1 1/2 minutes or until eggs are set. Cook a few seconds longer for firmer eggs.

Exchanges
1 Starch
5 Very Lean Meat

Calories	257
Calories from Fat	40
Total Fat	4 g
Saturated Fat	2 g
Cholesterol	10 mg
Sodium	761 mg
Carbohydrate	17 g
Dietary Fiber	2 g
Sugars	3 g
Protein	35 g

4. Place the cheese on half the omelet and fold the omelet in half. Slide out of the pan by tipping the pan and holding a plate vertically against the side of the pan. Invert the omelet onto the plate.
5. Cut in half and serve with toast.

Bran Cereal

Preparation time: **2 minutes**
Serves 2/Serving size: **1/2 recipe**

1 cup bran cereal
1 cup fat-free milk

Pour cereal into 2 bowls and pour milk on top.

Exchanges
2 Starch
1/2 Fat-Free Milk

Calories 167
  Calories from Fat . . 12
Total Fat. . . . . 1 g
  Saturated Fat. . . . . . 0 g
Cholesterol. . . . . 2 mg
Sodium . . . . 363 mg
Carbohydrate. . . . . 42 g
  Dietary Fiber . . . . . 18 g
  Sugars. . . . . 17 g
Protein. . . . . 8 g

SHOPPING LIST

Dairy
2 oz reduced-fat Swiss
  cheese

STAPLES

Rye bread
Cayenne pepper
Egg substitute
Olive oil cooking spray
Bran cereal
Fat-free milk
Salt
Black peppercorns

gorgonzola omelet

Gorgonzola Omelet
Bran Cereal

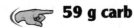 **59 g carb**

HELPFUL HINT

▍ Domestic crumbled Gorgonzola can be found in the dairy case of most supermarkets. You can use any type of blue cheese in this recipe.

COUNTDOWN

▍ Toast bread
▍ Make omelet
▍ Assemble cereal

Gorgonzola Omelet

Preparation time: **10 minutes**
Serves 2/Serving size: **1/2 recipe**

2 slices rye bread
　 Olive oil cooking spray
2 cups egg substitute
　 Pinch cayenne pepper
　 Salt and freshly ground black pepper to taste
1 oz crumbled Gorgonzola (1/3 cup)

1. Toast bread and spray one side of each slice with olive oil cooking spray. Set aside.
2. Pour egg substitute in a bowl and stir in cayenne pepper, salt, and pepper.
3. Heat a 9- or 10-inch nonstick skillet over medium-high heat and spray with cooking spray. Pour in egg mixture. Let the eggs set for about 30 seconds. Tip the pan and lightly move the eggs so that they all set. Cook 1 1/2 minutes or until eggs are set. Cook a few seconds longer for firmer eggs.

Exchanges
1 Starch
4 Very Lean Meat
1/2 Fat

Calories 237
　 Calories from Fat . . 45
Total Fat. . . . . 5 g
　 Saturated Fat. . . . . . 3 g
Cholesterol. . . . . . . 11 mg
Sodium. . . . . 829 mg
Carbohydrate. . . . . 17 g
　 Dietary Fiber . . . . . . 2 g
　 Sugars. . . . . 3 g
Protein. . . . . 29 g

4. Place the cheese on half the omelet and fold the omelet in half. Slide out of the pan by tipping the pan and holding a plate vertically against the side of the pan. Invert the omelet onto the plate.
5. Cut in half and serve with toast.

Bran Cereal

Preparation time: **2 minutes**
Serves 2/Serving size: **1/2 recipe**

1 cup bran cereal
1 cup fat-free milk

Pour cereal into 2 bowls and pour milk on top.

Exchanges
2 Starch
1/2 Fat-Free Milk

Calories 167
  Calories from Fat . . 12
Total Fat. . . . . 1 g
  Saturated Fat. . . . . . 0 g
Cholesterol. . . . . 2 mg
Sodium . . . . 363 mg
Carbohydrate. . . . . 42 g
  Dietary Fiber . . . . . 18 g
  Sugars. . . . . 17 g
Protein. . . . . 8 g

SHOPPING LIST

Dairy
2 oz crumbled
  Gorgonzola cheese

STAPLES

Rye bread
Cayenne pepper
Egg substitute
Olive oil cooking spray
Bran cereal
Fat-free milk
Salt
Black peppercorns

spinach omelet

Spinach and Mushroom Omelet
Bran Cereal

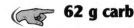 **62 g carb**

HELPFUL HINTS

▌ If you do not have a microwave oven, place the
spinach in a saucepan without water, cover,
and cook 3–4 minutes. Drain and add mushrooms, then sauté 1 minute.

▌ If mushroom slices are large, cut them in half.

COUNTDOWN

▌ Make filling
▌ Toast bread
▌ Complete omelet
▌ Assemble cereal

Spinach and Mushroom Omelet

Preparation time: **10 minutes**
Serves 2/serving size: **1/2 recipe**

  1 cup washed ready-to-eat spinach
1 1/2 cups sliced portobello mushrooms (1/4 lb)
  1/8 tsp nutmeg
  2 slices rye bread
    Olive oil cooking spray
  2 cups egg substitute
    Salt and freshly ground black pepper to taste

1. Place spinach and mushrooms in a
microwave-safe bowl. Sprinkle with nutmeg
and microwave on high for 3 minutes.

2. Toast bread and spray one side of each slice
with olive oil cooking spray. Set aside.

3. Pour egg substitute into a bowl and add salt
and pepper.

Exchanges
1 Starch
3 Very Lean Meat
1 Vegetable

Calories	205
Calories from Fat . .	11
Total Fat.	1 g
Saturated Fat.	0 g
Cholesterol.	0 mg
Sodium.	646 mg
Carbohydrate.	20 g
Dietary Fiber	3 g
Sugars.	3 g
Protein.	28 g

4. Heat a 9- or 10-inch nonstick skillet over medium-high heat and spray with cooking spray. Pour in egg mixture and let eggs set for 30 seconds. Tip the pan and lightly move the eggs so that they all set. Cook 1 1/2 minutes or until eggs are set. Cook a few seconds longer for firmer eggs.

5. Place spinach mixture on half the omelet and fold the omelet in half. Slide out of the pan by tipping the pan and holding a plate vertically against the side of the pan. Invert the omelet onto the plate.

6. Cut in half and serve with toast.

Bran Cereal

Preparation time: **2 minutes**
Serves 2/Serving size: **1/2 recipe**

1 cup bran cereal
1 cup fat-free milk

Pour cereal into 2 bowls and pour milk on top.

Exchanges
2 Starch
1/2 Fat-Free Milk

Calories 167
  Calories from Fat . . 12
Total Fat. . . . . 1 g
  Saturated Fat. . . . . . 0 g
Cholesterol. . . . . . . 2 mg
Sodium . . . . 363 mg
Carbohydrate. . . . . 42 g
  Dietary Fiber . . . . . 18 g
  Sugars. . . . . 17 g
Protein. . . . . 8 g

SHOPPING LIST

Produce
1 bag washed ready-to-eat spinach
1/4 lb portobello mushrooms

Grocery
Ground nutmeg

STAPLES

Egg substitute
Rye bread
Olive oil cooking spray
Bran cereal
Fat-free milk
Salt
Black peppercorns

smoked salmon omelet

Smoked Salmon Omelet
Bran Cereal 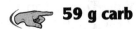 **59 g carb**

This is a great way to use leftover smoked salmon.

COUNTDOWN

▌ Toast bread
▌ Make omelet
▌ Assemble cereal

Smoked Salmon Omelet

Preparation time: **10 minutes**
Serves 2/serving size: **1/2 recipe**

2 slices rye bread
  Olive oil cooking spray
2 oz smoked salmon, cut into 1-inch pieces (1/3 cup)
2 Tbsp fat-free ricotta cheese
1 tsp dried dill
2 cups egg substitute
  Salt and freshly ground black pepper to taste

1. Toast bread and spray one side of each slice
   with olive oil cooking spray. Set aside.
2. Mix salmon, ricotta cheese, and dill together.
3. Pour egg substitute into a bowl and add salt
   and pepper.

Exchanges
1 Starch
4 Very Lean Meat

Calories 231
  Calories from Fat . . 19
Total Fat. . . . . 2 g
  Saturated Fat. . . . . . 0 g
Cholesterol. . . . . . . 12 mg
Sodium. . . . . 866 mg
Carbohydrate. . . . . 17 g
  Dietary Fiber . . . . . . 2 g
  Sugars. . . . . 3 g
Protein. . . . . 33 g

4. Heat a 9- or 10-inch nonstick skillet over medium-high heat and spray with cooking spray. Pour in egg mixture and let eggs set for 30 seconds. Tip the pan and lightly move the eggs so that they all set. Cook 1 1/2 minutes or until eggs are set. Cook a few seconds longer for firmer eggs.
5. Place the salmon mixture on half the omelet and fold the omelet in half. Slide out of the pan by tipping the pan and holding a plate vertically against the side of the pan. Invert the omelet onto the plate.
6. Cut in half and serve with toast.

Bran Cereal

Preparation time: **2 minutes**
Serves 2/Serving size: **1/2 recipe**

1 cup bran cereal
1 cup fat-free milk

Pour cereal into 2 bowls and pour milk on top.

Exchanges
2 Starch
1/2 Fat-Free Milk

Calories 167
   Calories from Fat . . 12
Total Fat. . . . . 1 g
   Saturated Fat. . . . . . 0 g
Cholesterol. . . . . 2 mg
Sodium . . . . 363 mg
Carbohydrate. . . . . 42 g
   Dietary Fiber . . . . . 18 g
   Sugars. . . . . 17 g
Protein. . . . . 8 g

SHOPPING LIST

Dairy
1 small carton fat-free
   ricotta cheese

Deli
2 oz smoked salmon

Grocery
Dried dill
1 small loaf rye bread

STAPLES

Egg substitute
Olive oil cooking spray
Bran cereal
Fat-free milk
Salt
Black peppercorns

breakfast egg sandwich

Breakfast Egg Sandwich
Oatmeal

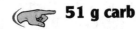 **51 g carb**

This is a quick egg dish that you can take on the run. You can make the egg the night before and assemble the sandwich the next morning.

HELPFUL HINT

▌ To flip the cooked egg pancake over quickly, cut it in half and flip each side separately. Or, place the pan under a broiler for a few seconds to cook the top.

COUNTDOWN

▌ Make oatmeal
▌ Make eggs
▌ Toast bread
▌ Assemble sandwich

Breakfast Egg Sandwich

Preparation time: **15 minutes**
Serves 2/Serving size: **1 sandwich**

2 whole eggs
4 egg whites
2 oz lean ham, torn into bite-size pieces (1/2 cup)
Salt and freshly ground black pepper to taste
Olive oil cooking spray
4 slices whole-wheat bread

1. Whisk together whole eggs and egg whites.
2. Stir in ham, salt, and pepper.
3. Heat a medium nonstick skillet over medium heat, spray with cooking spray, and add the egg mixture. Let sit for 3 to 4 minutes without stirring. Flip eggs over and cook 30 seconds.
4. Toast bread and spray one side of each slice with cooking spray. Divide eggs in half. Fold each half in half to fit in between the two bread slices, sprayed sides in.

Exchanges
2 Starch
2 Lean Meat
1/2 Fat

Calories 291
  Calories from Fat . . 81
Total Fat. . . . . 9 g
  Saturated Fat. . . . . . 3 g
Cholesterol. . . . . . 229 mg
Sodium. . . . . 844 mg
Carbohydrate. . . . . 27 g
  Dietary Fiber . . . . . . 4 g
  Sugars. . . . . 4 g
Protein. . . . . 26 g

Oatmeal

Preparation time: **5 minutes**
Serves 2/Serving size: **1/2 cup**

2/3 cup oatmeal
1 cup water
1 cup fat-free milk

1. Place oatmeal in a microwave-safe bowl and add water.
2. Microwave on high 3 minutes.
3. Place in 2 bowls and serve with milk.

Exchanges
1 Starch
1/2 Fat-Free Milk

Calories 147
  Calories from Fat . . 17
Total Fat. . . . . 2 g
  Saturated Fat. . . . . . 0 g
Cholesterol. . . . . . . 2 mg
Sodium. . . . . 64 mg
Carbohydrate. . . . . 24 g
  Dietary Fiber . . . . . . 3 g
  Sugars. . . . . 6 g
Protein. . . . . 9 g

SANDWICHES 'N STUFF

SHOPPING LIST

Deli
1 small package lean ham

STAPLES

Eggs (6 needed)
Whole-wheat bread
Olive oil cooking spray
Oatmeal
Fat-free milk
Salt
Black peppercorns

spicy grilled cheese

**Spicy Grilled Cheese
and Tomato Sandwich
Oatmeal**

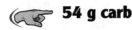 **54 g carb**

A creamy melted cheese sandwich with a hint of hot pepper and topped with sliced tomatoes is one of my husband's favorite quick breakfasts.

HELPFUL HINT

▌ You can use any type of reduced-fat cheese in this sandwich, but look for a brand that melts well.

COUNTDOWN

▌ Make oatmeal
▌ Make sandwich

Spicy Grilled Cheese and Tomato Sandwich

Preparation time: **10 minutes**
Serves 2/serving size: **1 sandwich**

3 oz sliced reduced-fat cheddar cheese
4 slices whole-wheat bread
2 tsp dry mustard
   Pinch cayenne pepper
1 small tomato, sliced

1. Place cheese on bread slices and sprinkle dry mustard and cayenne pepper on top.
2. Place tomato slices on top and toast in a toaster oven or place under a broiler for 1 minute or until cheese melts.

Exchanges
2 Starch
1 Medium-Fat Meat
1 Fat

Calories 277
   Calories from Fat . 108
Total Fat. . . . . 12 g
   Saturated Fat. . . . . . 5 g
Cholesterol. . . . . . 30 mg
Sodium. . . . . 661 mg
Carbohydrate. . . . . 30 g
   Dietary Fiber . . . . . . 5 g
   Sugars. . . . . 4 g
Protein. . . . . 17 g

Oatmeal

Preparation time: **5 minutes**
Serves 2/Serving size: **1/2 cup**

2/3 cup oatmeal
1 cup water
1 cup fat-free milk

1. Place oatmeal in a microwave-safe bowl and add water.
2. Microwave on high 3 minutes.
3. Place in 2 bowls and serve with milk.

Exchanges
1 Starch
1/2 Fat-Free Milk

Calories 147
  Calories from Fat . . 17
Total Fat . . . . 2 g
  Saturated Fat . . . . . . 0 g
Cholesterol . . . . 2 mg
Sodium . . . . 64 mg
Carbohydrate . . . . . 24 g
  Dietary Fiber . . . . . . 3 g
  Sugars . . . . 6 g
Protein . . . . 9 g

SHOPPING LIST

Produce
1 small tomato

Dairy
1 small package reduced-fat cheddar cheese

STAPLES

Dijon mustard
Cayenne pepper
Whole-wheat bread
Oatmeal
Fat-free milk

blueberry smoothie

Blueberry Smoothie
Tomato-Cheese Melt
Bran Cereal

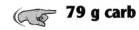 **79 g carb**

Rich, smooth, and easy to drink, smoothies are perfect for quick breakfasts. Many take-out smoothies are very high in carb. This one is not, takes only minutes to make, and tastes great!

HELPFUL HINTS

▌ You can use frozen or fresh blueberries in this recipe, but make sure the frozen ones are not packed in sugar syrup.

▌ If you use frozen blueberries, your smoothie may be very thick. Add a little water to thin.

▌ You can use any type of reduced-fat cheese in this sandwich, but look for a brand that melts well.

COUNTDOWN

▌ Make smoothie
▌ Make sandwich
▌ Assemble cereal

Blueberry Smoothie

Preparation time: **5 minutes**
Serves 2/serving size: **1/2 recipe**

1 cup blueberries
8 oz fat-free artificially sweetened blueberry yogurt
Sugar substitute equivalent to 2 tsp sugar
3 cups ice cubes

1. Place blueberries and yogurt in a blender and blend until smooth.
2. Add sugar substitute and ice and blend until thick.

Exchanges
1/2 Fruit
1 Fat-Free Milk

Calories 104
  Calories from Fat . . . 2
Total Fat. . . . . 0 g
  Saturated Fat. . . . . . 0 g
Cholesterol. . . . . 2 mg
Sodium. . . . . 64 mg
Carbohydrate. . . . . 22 g
  Dietary Fiber . . . . . . 2 g
  Sugars. . . . . 14 g
Protein. . . . . 4 g

Tomato-Cheese Melt

Preparation time: **5 minutes**
Serves 2/serving size: **1/2 recipe**

2 slices whole-wheat bread
2 Tbsp shredded reduced-fat cheddar cheese
1 small tomato, sliced

1. Sprinkle cheese on bread slices.
2. Top with tomato slices and place in toaster oven or under broiler for 2–3 minutes or until cheese melts.
3. Serve with smoothie.

Exchanges
1 Starch   1/2 Fat

Calories 100
  Calories from Fat . . 26
Total F tat . . . . 3 g
  Saturated Fat . . . . . . 1 g
Cholesterol . . . . 5 mg
Sodium . . . . 213 mg
Carbohydrate . . . . . 15 g
  Dietary Fiber . . . . . . 2 g
  Sugars . . . . 3 g
Protein . . . . 5 g

Bran Cereal

Preparation time: **2 minutes**
Serves 2/Serving size: **1/2 recipe**

1 cup bran cereal
1 cup fat-free milk

Pour cereal into 2 bowls and pour milk on top.

Exchanges
2 Starch   1/2 Fat-Free Milk

Calories 167
  Calories from Fat . . 12
Total Fat . . . . 1 g
  Saturated Fat . . . . . . 0 g
Cholesterol . . . . 2 mg
Sodium . . . . 363 mg
Carbohydrate . . . . . 42 g
  Dietary Fiber . . . . . 18 g
  Sugars . . . . 17 g
Protein . . . . 8 g

SHOPPING LIST

Produce
1 small carton
  blueberries or
  frozen blueberries
1 small tomato

Dairy
8 oz fat-free artificially sweetened
  blueberry yogurt
1 small package shredded
  reduced-fat cheddar cheese

STAPLES

Whole-wheat bread
Sugar substitute
Bran cereal
Fat-free milk

norwegian bagel

Norwegian Bagel Breakfast
Bran Cereal

 71 g carb

Bagels come in all sizes. For this recipe, choose ones that are about the size of a coffee can lid.

HELPFUL HINTS

▌ To quickly chop fresh dill, wash, dry, and snip the leaves with scissors right off the stem.
▌ If using dried dill, make sure the leaves are still green in the bottle for the best flavor. When they turn gray or brown, it's time for a new bottle.
▌ You can use smoked salmon in this recipe, but it's higher in fat than other smoked fish.

COUNTDOWN

▌ Assemble cereal
▌ Make bagel breakfast

Norwegian Bagel Breakfast

Preparation time: **5 minutes**
Serves 2/serving size: **1/2 recipe**

2 Tbsp fresh snipped dill (or 1 tsp dried dill)
2 tsp butter
1 small bagel (about 3 inches in diameter)
2 medium tomatoes, thinly sliced
1 medium cucumber, thinly sliced
6 oz smoked fish (white fish, haddock, or mackerel)
   Freshly ground black pepper to taste

Exchanges
1 Starch
3 Very Lean Meat
2 Vegetable
1 Fat

Calories 278
   Calories from Fat . . 52
Total Fat . . . . 6 g
   Saturated Fat . . . . . . 3 g
Cholesterol . . . . 75 mg
Sodium . . . . 893 mg
Carbohydrate . . . . . 29 g
   Dietary Fiber . . . . . . 3 g
   Sugars . . . . 8 g
Protein . . . . 27 g

1. Mix dill and butter together.
2. Slice bagel in half, spread with dill butter, and toast in toaster oven or under broiler.
3. Divide tomato slices, cucumber, and fish between 2 plates. Sprinkle with pepper.
4. Place one bagel half on each plate and serve.

Bran Cereal

Preparation time: **2 minutes**
Serves 2/Serving size: **1/2 recipe**

1 cup bran cereal
1 cup fat-free milk

Pour cereal into 2 bowls and pour milk on top.

Exchanges
2 Starch
1/2 Fat-Free Milk

Calories 167
 Calories from Fat . . 12
Total Fat. . . . . 1 g
 Saturated Fat. . . . . . 0 g
Cholesterol. . . . . 2 mg
Sodium . . . . 363 mg
Carbohydrate. . . . . 42 g
 Dietary Fiber . . . . . 18 g
 Sugars. . . . . 17 g
Protein. . . . . 8 g

SHOPPING LIST

Produce
2 medium tomatoes
1 medium cucumber
1 small bunch fresh dill
 (or dried dill)

Deli
6 oz smoked fish
 (white fish, haddock,
 salmon, or mackerel)

Grocery
1 small bagel

STAPLES

Butter
Black peppercorns
Bran cereal
Fat-free milk

toasted turkey

Toasted Turkey Breakfast Sandwich
Bran Cereal

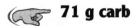 **71 g carb**

You can eat this 3-minute sandwich on the run! Or you can assemble it the night before and quickly toast or broil it the next morning.

COUNTDOWN

▌ Make sandwich
▌ Assemble cereal

Toasted Turkey Breakfast Sandwich

Preparation time: **5 minutes**
Serves 2/serving size: **1/2 recipe**

4 slices whole-wheat bread
1 Tbsp mayonnaise
1/2 lb sliced smoked turkey breast
1 cucumber, peeled and sliced (1 cup)
Salt and freshly ground black pepper to taste

1. Spread bread with mayonnaise. Divide turkey slices into four portions. Place one portion on each bread slice.
2. Toast in toaster oven or under broiler for 1–2 minutes.
3. Remove and place cucumber slices on top of 2 slices of bread. Sprinkle with salt and pepper and serve.

Exchanges
2 Starch
3 Lean Meat

Calories 314
Calories from Fat . . 79
Total Fat. . . . . 9 g
Saturated Fat. . . . . . 2 g
Cholesterol. . . . . . . 64 mg
Sodium. . . . . 1435 mg
Carbohydrate. . . . . 29 g
Dietary Fiber . . . . . . 4 g
Sugars. . . . . 5 g
Protein. . . . . 28 g

Bran Cereal

Preparation time: **2 minutes**
Serves 2/Serving size: **1/2 recipe**

1 cup bran cereal
1 cup fat-free milk

Pour cereal into 2 bowls and pour milk on top.

Exchanges
2 Starch
1/2 Fat-Free Milk

Calories 167
  Calories from Fat . . 12
Total Fat. . . . . 1 g
  Saturated Fat. . . . . . 0 g
Cholesterol. . . . . 2 mg
Sodium . . . . 363 mg
Carbohydrate. . . . . 42 g
  Dietary Fiber . . . . . 18 g
  Sugars. . . . . 17 g
Protein. . . . . 8 g

SHOPPING LIST

Produce
1 medium cucumber

Deli
1/2 lb sliced smoked turkey breast

STAPLES

Whole-wheat bread
Mayonnaise
Bran cereal
Fat-free milk
Salt
Black peppercorns

french toast

Nutty Cinnamon French Toast
Oatmeal

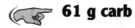 **61 g carb**

Sweet cinnamon and crunchy almonds top this easy
French toast.

COUNTDOWN

▌ Make oatmeal
▌ Make French toast

Nutty Cinnamon French Toast

Prep time: **15 minutes**
Serves 2/Serving size: **2 slices**

1 cup egg substitute
2 tsp sugar, divided
1 tsp cinnamon
1/4 cup slivered almonds
2 tsp canola oil
4 slices whole-wheat bread

1. Mix egg substitute and 1 tsp sugar together
   in a medium bowl. In a separate small bowl,
   mix 1 tsp sugar, cinnamon, and almonds.
2. Heat oil in a large nonstick skillet over
   medium heat. Dip bread in egg mixture,
   turning to coat both sides.
3. Cook French toast 1 minute and turn.
   Sprinkle cinnamon mixture on cooked side
   of bread.
4. Cover skillet with a lid and cook 2 minutes.

Exchanges
2 1/2 Starch
2 Very Lean Meat
2 Fat

Calories 350
  Calories from Fat . 136
Total Fat. . . . . 15 g
  Saturated Fat. . . . . . 1 g
Cholesterol. . . . . 0 mg
Sodium. . . . . 527 mg
Carbohydrate. . . . . 37 g
  Dietary Fiber . . . . . . 7 g
  Sugars. . . . . 8 g
Protein. . . . . 20 g

Oatmeal

Preparation time: **5 minutes**
Serves 2/Serving size: **1/2 cup**

2/3 cup oatmeal
 1 cup water
 1 cup fat-free milk

1. Place oatmeal in a microwave-safe bowl and add water.
2. Microwave on high 3 minutes.
3. Place in 2 bowls and serve with milk.

Exchanges
1 Starch
1/2 Fat-Free Milk

Calories 147
 Calories from Fat . . 17
Total Fat. . . . . 2 g
 Saturated Fat. . . . . . 0 g
Cholesterol. . . . . . . 2 mg
Sodium. . . . . 64 mg
Carbohydrate. . . . . 24 g
 Dietary Fiber . . . . . . 3 g
 Sugars. . . . . 6 g
Protein. . . . . 9 g

SHOPPING LIST

Grocery
1 small package slivered almonds

STAPLES

Egg substitute
Sugar
Ground cinnamon
Canola oil
Whole-wheat bread
Oatmeal
Fat-free milk

lunch

ham salad

**Ham, Swiss, Apple,
and Spinach Salad**

 39 g carb

HELPFUL HINTS

▌ Ask for the ham to be cut in a thick slice that you can cut into cubes.

COUNTDOWN

▌ Prepare ingredients
▌ Assemble salad

Ham, Swiss, Apple, and Spinach Salad

Preparation time: **5 minutes**
Serves 2/Serving size: **1/2 recipe**

4 cups washed ready-to-eat baby spinach
1 medium Golden Delicious or other apple, sliced
2 Tbsp Paul Newman's Oil and Balsamic Vinegar Salad Dressing
1 oz reduced-fat Swiss cheese, torn into bite-sized pieces
6 oz lean ham cut into 1/2-inch cubes
1 medium tomato cut into small wedges
2 slices whole-wheat bread

1. Toss spinach and apple with dressing.
2. Sprinkle cheese and ham on top.
3. Arrange tomato wedges around edge.
4. Serve with bread.

Exchanges

1 Starch	1 Fruit
3 Lean Meat	1 Fat
1 Vegetable	

Calories 405
  Calories from Fat . 139
Total Fat. . . . . 15 g
  Saturated Fat. . . . . . 4 g
Cholesterol. . . . . . . 53 mg
Sodium. . . . . 1395 mg
Carbohydrate. . . . . 39 g
  Dietary Fiber . . . . . . 8 g
  Sugars. . . . . 20 g
Protein. . . . . 31 g

SALADS

SHOPPING LIST

Produce
1 bag washed ready-to-eat baby spinach
1 medium apple
1 medium tomato

Dairy
1 oz reduced-fat Swiss cheese
Deli
6 oz lean ham

STAPLES

Paul Newman's Oil and Balsamic Vinegar Salad Dressing
Whole-wheat bread

shrimp salad

Shrimp and Black-Eyed Pea Salad
Peaches

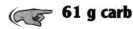 **61 g carb**

In the South, black-eyed pea salad is also known as Mississippi Caviar. I've added some cooked shrimp to make this quick lunch salad a more complete meal. Black-eyed peas are a small beige bean that have a black circle at their inner curve and were originally imported for livestock feed.

HELPFUL HINTS

▌ You can use frozen or canned black-eyed peas in this salad, but be sure to rinse the canned ones. I prefer to use frozen black-eyed peas. They have an excellent texture and flavor and work well in this recipe.
▌ Buy peeled, cooked shrimp from the seafood counter.
▌ You can use any type of lettuce.

COUNTDOWN

▌ Cook black-eyed peas
▌ Assemble salad
▌ Prepare fruit

Shrimp and Black-Eyed Pea Salad

Preparation time: **15 minutes**
Serves 2/Serving size: **1/2 recipe**

1 8-oz package frozen black-eyed peas (1 1/2 cups) or 1 1/2 cups canned black-eyed peas, rinsed and drained
2 Tbsp Paul Newman's Oil and Vinegar Salad Dressing
1/2 cup diced red onion
   Several drops hot pepper sauce
   Salt and freshly ground black pepper to taste
1/2 cup diced red bell pepper
6 oz peeled cooked shrimp
   Several red leaf lettuce leaves, rinsed and dried
2 slices whole-wheat bread

1. Bring a medium saucepan half filled with water to a boil. Add the black-eyed peas, cover with a lid, and cook 15 minutes or until the peas are soft. Or, place in a microwave-safe bowl with 2 Tbsp water and microwave on high 5 minutes. (Omit this step if using canned black-eyed peas.)
2. Place dressing in a medium mixing bowl and add onion, hot pepper sauce, salt, and pepper.
3. Drain black-eyed peas and add to dressing with red bell pepper and shrimp. Toss well. Taste for seasoning. Add more salt, pepper, or hot pepper sauce to taste.
4. Line 2 dinner plates with lettuce leaves and spoon salad on top.
5. Serve with bread.

Exchanges
3 Starch
3 Very Lean Meat
1 Vegetable
1 1/2 Fat

Calories	423
Calories from Fat	100
Total Fat	11 g
Saturated Fat	2 g
Cholesterol	165 mg
Sodium	430 mg
Carbohydrate	50 g
Dietary Fiber	10 g
Sugars	7 g
Protein	32 g

SALADS

Peaches

Serve 1 medium peach per person.

SHOPPING LIST

Produce
1 red bell pepper
1 small head red leaf lettuce
2 medium peaches

Seafood
6 oz peeled cooked shrimp

Grocery
1 8-oz package frozen black-eyed peas or 2 cans black-eyed peas

STAPLES

Red onion
Paul Newman's Oil and Vinegar Salad Dressing
Hot pepper sauce
Whole-wheat bread
Salt
Black peppercorns

tuscan bean salad

**Tuscan Bean and Tuna Salad
  with Tomatoes**
Watermelon Cubes

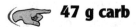 **47 g carb**

Vinaigrette dressing makes this popular Italian salad a nice
change from tuna salad with a mayonnaise base. The tomatoes
are a colorful complement.

HELPFUL HINTS

▌ You can use any type of canned bean in this
  salad.
▌ Buy the best quality white meat tuna packed
  in water for the tastiest results.
▌ You can find watermelon cubes in season in
  the produce section of most supermarkets.

COUNTDOWN

▌ Make salad

Tuscan Bean and Tuna Salad with Tomatoes

Preparation time: **10 minutes**
Serves 2/Serving size: **1/2 recipe**

  1 cup rinsed and drained small white beans (cannellini or navy)
1/4 cup diced red onion
  1 6-oz can white meat tuna packed in water
1/2 cup chopped fresh parsley, divided
  2 Tbsp plus 2 tsp Paul Newman's Oil and Balsamic Vinegar Salad
    Dressing
    Salt and freshly ground black pepper to taste
1/2 head red leaf lettuce
  2 cups tomatoes, cut into 1/2-inch pieces

1. Place beans in a serving bowl and add onion.
2. Drain tuna and break into large flakes. Add to the beans.
3. Add half the parsley, 2 Tbsp dressing, and salt and pepper to taste. Gently toss.
4. Arrange lettuce leaves on a serving platter and spoon salad over the leaves.
5. Toss tomatoes with 2 tsp dressing, add salt and pepper to taste, and toss again.
6. Arrange tomatoes around edges of salad plate.
7. Sprinkle tuna and tomatoes with the remaining parsley and serve.

Exchanges
1 1/2 Starch
3 Very Lean Meat
2 Vegetable
1 Fat

Calories 352
  Calories from Fat . . 72
Total Fat. . . . . 8 g
  Saturated Fat. . . . . . 1 g
Cholesterol. . . . . . 21 mg
Sodium. . . . . 612 mg
Carbohydrate. . . . . 36 g
  Dietary Fiber . . . . . 10 g
  Sugars. . . . . 8 g
Protein. . . . . 30 g

Watermelon Cubes

Serve 1 cup per person.

SHOPPING LIST

Produce
1 red onion
1 small bunch parsley
1 small head red leaf
  lettuce
2 medium tomatoes
1 small container
  watermelon cubes
  (about 2 cups)

Grocery
1 6-oz can white meat
  tuna packed in water
1 8-oz can white beans
  (cannellini or navy)

STAPLES

Paul Newman's Oil and
  Balsamic Vinegar
  Salad Dressing
Salt
Black peppercorns

antipasto platter

Antipasto Platter
Seedless Grapes

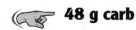 **48 g carb**

"Little bites," whether they're Spanish tapas, Mediterranean mezze, or Italian antipasto, are always colorful and enticing. Here's a quick antipasto platter that can be assembled in just a few minutes. It's great for a weekend lunch or for guests.

HELPFUL HINTS

▌ Look for low-fat meats in the deli to vary the recipe given.
▌ Pepperoncini are small, hot peppers that can be bought in a jar or can.
▌ You can add any type of vegetables to the platter.

COUNTDOWN

▌ Warm rolls
▌ Assemble platter

Antipasto Platter

Preparation time: **10 minutes**
Serves 2/Serving size: **1/2 recipe**

1/2 head red leaf lettuce leaves (about 3 cups)
2 oz sliced lean ham (about 1/2 cup)
2 oz roasted chicken breast slices (about 1/2 cup)
2 oz part-skim mozzarella cheese, sliced (scant 1/2 cup)
2 cups canned or jarred roasted red peppers
1/2 cup canned or jarred marinated artichoke quarters (6.5 oz jar), drained
8 pitted black olives
2 small whole-wheat rolls (about 1 1/4 oz per roll)

1. Preheat oven or toaster oven to 300°F.
2. Wash and dry lettuce leaves and place on 2 plates. Place rolls in oven.
3. Starting in the center, arrange ham slices overlapping each other in a line towards the edge of the plate. Arrange a line of chicken on opposite side of the plate. Similarly, arrange a line of mozzarella so that you have three lines radiating from the center of the plate.
4. Fill in the rest of the plate with the remaining vegetables and olives.
5. Serve with warm rolls.

Exchanges
1 Starch
3 Lean Meat
4 Vegetable
1/2 Fat

Calories 368
  Calories from Fat . 114
Total Fat. . . . . 13 g
  Saturated Fat. . . . . . 4 g
Cholesterol. . . . . . 56 mg
Sodium. . . . . 1010 mg
Carbohydrate. . . . . 34 g
  Dietary Fiber . . . . . . 7 g
  Sugars. . . . . 7 g
Protein. . . . . 29 g

SALADS

Seedless Grapes

Serve 1/2 cup per person.

SHOPPING LIST

Produce
1 head red leaf lettuce
1 large bunch seedless grapes

Dairy
2 oz part-skim mozzarella cheese

Deli
2 oz low-fat ham
2 oz roasted chicken

Grocery
1 jar roasted red peppers
1 can or jar marinated artichokes
1 can or jar pitted black olives
2 small whole-wheat rolls

shrimp caesar salad

Shrimp Caesar Salad
Kiwis

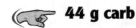 **44 g carb**

Succulent shrimp and romaine lettuce are the base for this tasty
Caesar salad.

HELPFUL HINTS

- Buy peeled, cooked shrimp from the seafood
  counter.
- Buy good-quality Parmesan cheese and ask
  the market to grate it for you or chop it in the
  food processor. Freeze extra for quick use.
  You can spoon out the quantity you need and
  leave the rest frozen.

COUNTDOWN

- Warm bread
- Assemble salad
- Prepare fruit

Shrimp Caesar Salad

Preparation time: **5 minutes**
Serves 2/Serving size: **1/2 recipe**

2 whole-wheat pita breads
4 cups washed ready-to-eat Romaine lettuce
6 oz peeled cooked medium shrimp
2 Tbsp Caesar salad dressing
2 Tbsp grated Parmesan cheese
  Freshly ground black pepper to taste

1. Preheat oven or toaster oven to 300°F.
2. Place lettuce and shrimp in a bowl and toss with dressing. Place pita bread in oven.
3. Divide salad between 2 plates. Sprinkle Parmesan on top and add pepper.
4. Serve with warm pita bread.

Exchanges
2 Starch
3 Very Lean Meat
1 1/2 Fat

Calories 337
  Calories from Fat . 106
Total Fat. . . . . 12 g
  Saturated Fat. . . . . . 2 g
Cholesterol. . . . . 172 mg
Sodium. . . . . 517 mg
Carbohydrate. . . . . 33 g
  Dietary Fiber . . . . . . 2 g
  Sugars. . . . . 4 g
Protein. . . . . 27 g

Kiwis

Serve 1 kiwi per person.

SALADS

SHOPPING LIST

Produce
1 bag washed ready-to-eat Romaine lettuce
2 medium kiwis

Seafood
6 oz peeled cooked medium shrimp

Grocery
2 whole-wheat pita breads
1 bottle Caesar dressing

STAPLES

Parmesan cheese
Black peppercorns

smoked fish salad

Smoked Fish Salad
Fruit-Flavored Yogurt

☞ **57 g carb**

Smoked fish, onions, and dill pickles is a typical English pub lunch. I have combined these ingredients into a quick and tasty lunch salad.

HELPFUL HINTS

- Choose any type of smoked white fish (haddock, amberjack, kingfish, or mackerel).
- To cut onion rings, slice the onion parallel to the root in 1/2-inch slices.

COUNTDOWN

- Blanch onion rings
- Assemble salad
- Make toast

Smoked Fish Salad

Preparation time: **10 minutes**
Serves 2/Serving size: **1/2 recipe**

- **1** medium onion, sliced into rings (1 cup)
- **1/2** lb smoked white fish, all bones removed
- **2** Tbsp Paul Newman's Oil and Vinegar Salad Dressing
- **1/2** cup sliced dill pickles
- **4** slices rye bread

1. Bring a small saucepan half filled with water to a boil. Add sliced onion rings. When water returns to a boil, drain and run rings under cold water.
2. Cut fish into pieces about 2 inches long and 1 inch wide. Place smoked fish in a shallow dish or bowl and spread onion rings on top.
3. Spoon dressing over fish and onion rings.
4. Slice pickles on the diagonal and arrange around edge of plate.
5. Toast bread and serve with salad.

Exchanges
2 Starch
3 Very Lean Meat
1 Vegetable
2 Fat

Calories 379
Calories from Fat . . 99
Total Fat . . . . 11 g
Saturated Fat . . . . . . 2 g
Cholesterol . . . . . . 87 mg
Sodium . . . . 1655 mg
Carbohydrate . . . . . 34 g
Dietary Fiber . . . . . . 5 g
Sugars . . . . 8 g
Protein . . . . 34 g

Fruit-Flavored Yogurt

Serve 1 8-oz carton fat-free artificially sweetened fruit-flavored yogurt per person.

SHOPPING LIST

Produce
1 medium onion

Dairy
2 8-oz cartons fat-free artificially sweetened fruit-flavored yogurt

Deli
1/2 lb smoked white fish

Grocery
1 small jar dill pickles
1 small loaf rye bread

STAPLES

Paul Newman's Oil and Vinegar Salad Dressing

turkey salad

Smoked Turkey Waldorf Salad
Tangerines

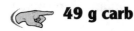 **49 g carb**

Crunchy apples, celery, and walnuts mixed with smoked turkey make a crisp lunch salad.

HELPFUL HINTS

▌ Look for smoked turkey breast in the deli department. Ask for the turkey to be cut in one thick slice that you can make into cubes.
▌ If you prefer, you can use smoked chicken breast or roast chicken.

COUNTDOWN

▌ Make salad
▌ Toast bread

Smoked Turkey Waldorf Salad

Preparation time: **10 minutes**
Serves 2/Serving size: **1/2 recipe**

2 Tbsp reduced-fat mayonnaise
2 Tbsp lemon juice
 Salt and freshly ground black pepper to taste
2 celery stalks, sliced (1 cup)
2 small red apples, cored and cut into 1/2-inch cubes (2 cups)
1 Tbsp broken walnuts (1/4 oz)
1/2 lb smoked turkey breast cut into 1/2-inch cubes
 Several romaine lettuce leaves, washed and dried
2 slices whole-wheat bread

1. Mix mayonnaise and lemon juice together in a medium bowl. Add salt and pepper.
2. Toss celery, apples, walnuts, and turkey in the mayonnaise. Taste for seasoning and add more salt and pepper, if needed.
3. Place lettuce leaves on 2 dinner plates and spoon salad onto leaves.
4. Toast bread and serve with salad.

Exchanges
1 Starch
3 Very Lean Meat
1 1/2 Fruit
1 1/2 Fat

Calories 354
 Calories from Fat . . 88
Total Fat . . . . 10 g
 Saturated Fat . . . . . . 2 g
Cholesterol . . . . 65 mg
Sodium . . . . 1427 mg
Carbohydrate . . . . . 40 g
 Dietary Fiber . . . . . . 7 g
 Sugars . . . . 20 g
Protein . . . . 27 g

Tangerines

Serve 1 medium tangerine per person.

SHOPPING LIST

Produce
1 lemon
1 small head Romaine lettuce
1 bag celery
2 small red apples
2 medium tangerines

Deli
1/2 lb smoked turkey breast

Grocery
1 small package broken walnuts

STAPLES

Reduced-fat mayonnaise
Whole-wheat bread
Salt
Black peppercorns

peasant salad

Italian Peasant Salad
Plums

 50 g carb

A colorful array of vegetables—blanched, dressed, and topped with coarsely chopped eggs—is a tasty salad served in Northern Italy. The vegetables are cooked separately in a microwave oven.

HELPFUL HINTS

▌ Buy peeled baby carrots—they're so easy to use.
▌ You can serve the vegetables raw instead of cooked.
▌ You can use any type of lettuce.
▌ You can cook the eggs in advance and keep them several days in the refrigerator

COUNTDOWN

▌ Cook eggs
▌ Cook vegetables
▌ Assemble salad

Italian Peasant Salad

Preparation time: **15 minutes**
Serves 2/Serving size: **1/2 recipe**

  6 eggs
1/2 lb green beans, trimmed (2 cups)
1/2 lb peeled baby carrots (2 cups)
1/4 lb broccoli florets (2 cups)
  2 Tbsp Paul Newman's Oil and Balsamic Vinegar Salad Dressing, divided
    Several leaves Boston lettuce
1/2 cup arugula, torn into small bite-sized pieces
  2 slices whole-wheat bread

1. Place eggs in a small saucepan and cover with cold water. Place over medium-high heat and bring to a boil. Reduce heat to low and gently simmer 12 minutes.
2. Drain and fill the pan with cold water. When eggs are cool to the touch, peel and cut in half lengthwise. Remove the yolks from 4 of the eggs and discard.
3. Coarsely chop the 6 egg whites and 2 yolks. Set aside.
4. Place beans, carrots, and broccoli in 3 separate bowls. Cook each vegetable in a microwave oven on high for 2 minutes.
5. Place vegetables in a medium mixing bowl and toss with 1 Tbsp dressing.
6. Place lettuce leaves on 2 plates and arrange vegetables in the center.
7. Sprinkle coarsely chopped eggs on top of the vegetables, sprinkle with arugula, and drizzle remaining dressing over the salad.
8. Serve with bread or toast.

Exchanges
1 Starch
1 Lean Meat
5 Vegetable
1 1/2 Fat

Calories 332
  Calories from Fat . 104
Total Fat . . . . 12 g
  Saturated Fat . . . . . . 3 g
Cholesterol . . . . . . 213 mg
Sodium . . . . 563 mg
Carbohydrate . . . . . 40 g
  Dietary Fiber . . . . . 11 g
  Sugars . . . . 13 g
Protein . . . . 21 g

SALADS

Plums

Serve 1 medium plum per person.

SHOPPING LIST

Produce
1/2 lb green beans
1/2 lb peeled baby carrots
1/4 lb broccoli
1 small head Boston lettuce
1 small bunch arugula
2 medium plums

STAPLES

Eggs (6 needed)
Whole-wheat bread
Paul Newman's Oil and Balsamic
  Vinegar Salad Dressing

chicken salad

Toasted Almond Chicken Salad
Pineapple Chunks

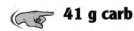 **41 g carb**

Chicken salad is easy to make using ready-to-eat cooked
chicken pieces.

HELPFUL HINTS

▌ Look for ready-to-eat roasted chicken strips in
the cooked meat section or in the refrigerated
ready-to-eat meat cases of the supermarket.
▌ If you do not have a toaster oven, toast
almonds in a small skillet over medium heat
for about 30 seconds or until golden.
▌ You can find fresh pineapple chunks in the
produce section of the supermarket.

COUNTDOWN

▌ Make salad

Toasted Almond Chicken Salad

Preparation time: **5 minutes**
Serves 2/Serving size: **1/2 recipe**

8 oz ready-to-eat roasted chicken strips
2 stalks celery, sliced (2 cups)
1 Tbsp slivered almonds
2 Tbsp reduced-fat mayonnaise
1 tsp dried dill
    Salt and freshly ground black pepper to taste
2 large slices rye bread

1. Coarsely chop chicken and celery in a food processor or by hand. Remove to a bowl.
2. Toast almonds in a toaster oven until golden.
3. Add almonds to chicken and stir in mayonnaise, dill, salt, and pepper.
4. Spoon salad onto two plates and serve with bread or toast.

Exchanges
1 Starch
5 Very Lean Meat
1 Vegetable
2 Fat

Calories 365
  Calories from Fat . 111
Total Fat. . . . . 12 g
  Saturated Fat. . . . . . 2 g
Cholesterol. . . . . . 101 mg
Sodium. . . . . 524 mg
Carbohydrate. . . . . 22 g
  Dietary Fiber . . . . . . 5 g
  Sugars. . . . . 2 g
Protein. . . . . 40 g

Pineapple Chunks

Serve 1 cup per person.

SHOPPING LIST

STAPLES

Produce
1 package fresh
  pineapple chunks

Meat
1/2 lb ready-to-eat
  roasted chicken strips

Grocery
1 small package sliced
  almonds
1 small loaf rye bread
1 bottle dried dill

Reduced-fat mayonnaise
Celery
Salt
Black peppercorns

salsa beef

Salsa Beef Salad
Oranges

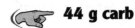 **44 g carb**

Roast beef, salsa, shredded lettuce, and cheese give this salad the hearty flavors of the Southwest.

HELPFUL HINTS

▌ Buy salsa that has no added sugar or oil.
▌ Ask for sliced lean roast beef in the deli section of the supermarket.
▌ You can use shredded, reduced-fat Mexican-style cheese instead of Monterey Jack.

COUNTDOWN

▌ Prepare ingredients
▌ Assemble salad

Salsa Beef Salad

Preparation time: **5 minutes**
Serves 2/Serving size: **1/2 recipe**

6 oz sliced lean roast beef
5 cups shredded lettuce
1/4 cup tomato salsa
2 Tbsp Paul Newman's Oil and Vinegar Salad Dressing
1/2 cup frozen corn kernels
2 Tbsp shredded reduced-fat Monterey Jack cheese
2 medium seven-grain dinner rolls

1. Preheat oven or toaster oven to 300°F.
2. Slice beef into 2-inch strips. Arrange lettuce on a serving platter and place beef strips on top. Place rolls in oven.
3. Mix salsa with dressing and spoon over salad.
4. Defrost corn in microwave oven on high 1 minute.
5. Sprinkle corn and cheese on top of salad and serve with rolls.

Exchanges
2 Starch
3 Lean Meat
1 Vegetable
1 1/2 Fat

Calories 413
  Calories from Fat . 140
Total Fat. . . . . 16 g
  Saturated Fat. . . . . . 4 g
Cholesterol. . . . . . . 59 mg
Sodium. . . . . 863 mg
Carbohydrate. . . . . 36 g
  Dietary Fiber . . . . . . 5 g
  Sugars. . . . . 6 g
Protein. . . . . 31 g

SALADS

Oranges

Serve 1 medium orange per person.

SHOPPING LIST

Produce
1 head lettuce or 1 bag washed shredded ready-to-eat lettuce
2 medium oranges

Dairy
1 small package shredded reduced-fat Monterey Jack cheese

Deli
6 oz sliced lean roast beef

Grocery
1 small jar tomato salsa
1 small package frozen corn kernels
1 package seven-grain dinner rolls

STAPLES

Paul Newman's Oil and Vinegar Salad Dressing

chef's salad

Chef's Salad
Apples

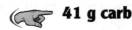 **41 g carb**

A salad of julienne slices of turkey, ham, cheese, and vegetables served on a crisp bed of lettuce and topped with dressing has been an American staple for nearly 100 years. Over time the ingredients have changed a little, but the style of this classic remains the same. Here is a simple, quick version.

HELPFUL HINTS

▌ You can prepare these vegetables in a food processor with either a julienne or a slicing blade.
▌ Buy turkey and ham that are not honey baked and do not have added sugar.

COUNTDOWN

▌ Prepare ingredients
▌ Assemble salad

Chef's Salad

Preparation time: **5 minutes**
Serves 2/Serving size: **1/2 recipe**

4 cups washed ready-to-eat lettuce
3 oz smoked turkey breast, cut in julienne slices (about 3/4 cup)
2 oz low-fat ham, cut in julienne slices (about 1/2 cup)
1 oz reduced-fat cheddar cheese, cut in julienne slices (scant 1/4 cup)
1/2 cucumber, peeled and cut in julienne slices (about 1 1/4 cup)
1 small green bell pepper, seeded and cut in julienne slices (about 2 cups)
1 medium tomato, quartered
2 Tbsp Paul Newman's Oil and Vinegar Salad Dressing
2 slices whole-wheat bread

1. Place the lettuce on a platter.
2. Arrange turkey, ham, cheese, cucumber, green pepper, and tomato in pie-shaped wedges over the lettuce.
3. Drizzle dressing over vegetables.
4. Serve with bread.

Exchanges
1 Starch
2 Lean Meat
2 Vegetable
1 1/2 Fat

Calories 322
  Calories from Fat . 132
Total Fat . . . . 15 g
  Saturated Fat . . . . . . 4 g
Cholesterol . . . . 48 mg
Sodium . . . . 1152 mg
Carbohydrate . . . . . 25 g
  Dietary Fiber . . . . . . 5 g
  Sugars . . . . 9 g
Protein . . . . 24 g

SALADS

Apples

Serve 1 small apple per person.

SHOPPING LIST

Produce
1 bag washed ready-to-eat lettuce
1 medium cucumber
1 small green bell pepper
1 medium tomato
2 small apples

Deli
3 oz smoked turkey breast
2 oz low-fat ham

Dairy
1 oz reduced-fat cheddar cheese

STAPLES

Paul Newman's Oil and Vinegar Salad Dressing
Whole-wheat bread

tangy chicken salad

Tangy Chicken and Pear Salad
Fresh Blueberries

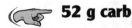 **52 g carb**

Chicken and sweet juicy pears blend with spicy horseradish to make a tangy lunch salad.

COUNTDOWN

▌ Prepare ingredients
▌ Assemble salad
▌ Toast bread

Tangy Chicken and Pear Salad

Preparation time: **5 minutes**
Serves 2/Serving size: **1/2 recipe**

- **2** Tbsp reduced-fat mayonnaise
- **2** Tbsp horseradish
- **2** Tbsp Dijon mustard
- **1** Tbsp lime or lemon juice
- **1** ripe pear, cored and cut into 1/2-inch pieces, skin left on (1/2 cup)
- **1/2** lb roasted boneless skinless rotisserie chicken breast, cubed
- **8** Romaine lettuce leaves, washed
- **4** tablespoons chopped fresh chives
- **2** slices whole-wheat bread

1. Mix mayonnaise, horseradish, mustard, and lime or lemon juice together in a salad bowl. Add pear and chicken.
2. Place lettuce leaves on 2 plates. Spoon salad on top and sprinkle chives on salad.
3. Toast bread and serve with salad.

Exchanges

1 Starch
5 Very Lean Meat
1 Fruit
1 1/2 Fat

Calories 390
  Calories from Fat . 102
Total Fat . . . . 11 g
  Saturated Fat . . . . . . 2 g
Cholesterol . . . . . . 101 mg
Sodium . . . . 764 mg
Carbohydrate . . . . . 32 g
  Dietary Fiber . . . . . . 5 g
  Sugars . . . . 15 g
Protein . . . . 41 g

SALADS

Fresh Blueberries

Serve 1 cup per person.

SHOPPING LIST

Produce
1 lime or lemon
1 small head Romaine
  lettuce
1 ripe pear
1 small bunch chives
1/2 pint fresh
  blueberries

Deli
1/2 lb roasted chicken
  breast

Grocery
1 small jar horseradish

STAPLES

Reduced-fat mayonnaise
Dijon mustard
Whole-wheat bread

hero sandwich

Italian Hero Sandwich
Grapefruit

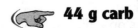 **44 g carb**

Heros, submarines, hoagies—call them what you like. These American sandwiches are bigger than life! This one is easy to make and doesn't break your carb budget.

HELPFUL HINTS

▌ Use any type of lean deli meat in this sandwich.
▌ You can add fresh arugula and basil if you like.

COUNTDOWN

▌ Prepare ingredients
▌ Assemble sandwich

Italian Hero Sandwich

Preparation time: **5 minutes**
Serves 2/Serving size: **1/2 recipe**

2 small French or Italian whole-grain rolls (about 2 oz each)
  Olive oil cooking spray
2 plum tomatoes, thinly sliced
4 oz roasted chicken breast pieces (1 cup)
2 oz part-skim mozzarella cheese, sliced (1/2 cup)
1 cup canned pimientos, drained and cut into strips
  Salt and freshly ground black pepper to taste

1. Slice rolls in half horizontally and remove the centers. Spray each side with cooking spray.
2. Layer tomato, chicken, and mozzarella on one side of the roll. Add pimientos, salt, and pepper.
3. Cover with top of roll, cut in half, and serve.

Exchanges
2 Starch
3 Very Lean Meat
1 Vegetable
1 Fat

Calories 326
  Calories from Fat . . 73
Total Fat. . . . . 8 g
  Saturated Fat. . . . . . 4 g
Cholesterol. . . . . . . 63 mg
Sodium. . . . . 507 mg
Carbohydrate. . . . . 31 g
  Dietary Fiber . . . . . . 4 g
  Sugars. . . . . 7 g
Protein. . . . . 30 g

Grapefruit

Serve 1/2 large grapefruit per person.

SHOPPING LIST

Produce
2 plum tomatoes
1 large grapefruit

Dairy
1 small package part-skim mozzarella cheese

Deli
4 oz roasted chicken breast pieces

Grocery
2 small French or Italian whole-grain rolls (about 2 oz each)
1 small can pimientos

STAPLES

Olive oil cooking spray
Salt
Black peppercorns

grilled turkey sausage

Grilled Turkey Sausage
   with Mustard and
     Sweet Pickle Relish
Fresh Strawberries

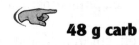 **48 g carb**

Grilled turkey sausages with mustard and pickle relish make a delicious change from traditional hot dogs. There are several different flavors of low-fat turkey sausages available. They come spicy or mild, smoked or plain. Pick your favorite for this tasty lunch.

HELPFUL HINT

▌ If you can't find whole-wheat hot dog buns, use 2 slices of whole-wheat bread instead.

COUNTDOWN

▌ Cook sausages
▌ Assemble sandwich

Grilled Turkey Sausage with Mustard and Sweet Pickle Relish

Preparation time: **15 minutes**
Serves 2/Serving size: **1/2 recipe**

  Olive oil cooking spray
2 low-fat turkey sausages (1/2 pound)
2 whole-wheat hot dog buns
1 Tbsp mustard
2 Tbsp sweet pickle relish
2 medium tomatoes, sliced

1. Heat a stovetop grill over medium-high heat. Spray grill with cooking spray. Grill sausages 8–10 minutes, turning to make sure all sides are cooked.
2. While sausages cook, open hot dog buns and toast on grill for 2 minutes.
3. Spread mustard on buns. Add sausage and spoon relish on top.
4. Serve sliced tomatoes on the side.

Exchanges
1/2 Carbohydrate
1 1/2 Starch
2 Lean Meat
1 Vegetable
1 Fat

Calories 329
 Calories from Fat . 107
Total Fat. . . . . 12 g
 Saturated Fat. . . . . . 3 g
Cholesterol. . . . . . . 72 mg
Sodium. . . . . 2166 mg
Carbohydrate. . . . . 37 g
 Dietary Fiber . . . . . . 7 g
 Sugars. . . . . 15 g
Protein. . . . . 22 g

Fresh Strawberries

Serve 1 cup per person.

SHOPPING LIST

STAPLES

Produce
2 medium tomatoes
1 pint fresh strawberries

Grocery
1 jar sweet pickle relish
1 package whole-wheat
  hot dog buns

Mustard
Olive oil cooking spray

Meat
1 small package low-fat
  turkey sausage

shrimp roll

**Shrimp Roll
Apples**

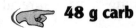 **48 g carb**

Shrimp tossed with homemade tartar sauce is a New England favorite. Drive along the coastline from Connecticut to Maine and you'll find little roadside stands selling lobster, shrimp, or clam rolls. This simple version captures their flavor.

HELPFUL HINTS

▌ Buy peeled, cooked shrimp from the seafood counter.
▌ If whole-wheat hot dog buns are not available, use 2 slices of whole-wheat bread.

COUNTDOWN

▌ Make filling
▌ Assemble sandwich

Shrimp Roll

Preparation time: **5 minutes**
Serves 2/Serving size: **1/2 recipe**

2 Tbsp mayonnaise
1 tsp Dijon mustard
1 Tbsp drained sweet pickle relish
   Salt and freshly ground black pepper to taste
1/2 lb peeled cooked shrimp
2 hot whole-wheat hot dog buns
1 cup washed shredded lettuce

1. Mix mayonnaise, mustard, and relish together in a medium bowl. Add salt and pepper.
2. Add shrimp and toss to coat.
3. Split hot dog rolls open and toast in a toaster oven or under a broiler.
4. Fill rolls with lettuce and shrimp mixture.

Exchanges
1 1/2 Starch
4 Very Lean Meat
1 1/2 Fat

Calories 319
  Calories from Fat . 121
Total Fat. . . . . 13 g
  Saturated Fat. . . . . . 2 g
Cholesterol. . . . . 229 mg
Sodium. . . . . 689 mg
Carbohydrate. . . . . 24 g
  Dietary Fiber . . . . . . 6 g
  Sugars. . . . . 4 g
Protein. . . . . 29 g

Apples

Serve 1 medium apple per person.

SHOPPING LIST

STAPLES

Produce
1 head lettuce or 1 bag washed shredded ready-to-eat lettuce
2 medium apples

Seafood
6 oz peeled cooked shrimp

Grocery
1 jar sweet pickle relish
2 whole-wheat hot dog buns

Mayonnaise
Dijon mustard
Salt
Black peppercorns

turkey wrap

Quick Turkey Wrap
Tangerines

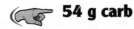 **54 g carb**

Turkey slices, sweet pimientos, and pickles rolled together in a soft tortilla make a colorful, quick sandwich that can be eaten on the run.

HELPFUL HINT

▌ This filling's also great in a whole-wheat pita pocket.

COUNTDOWN

▌ Prepare ingredients
▌ Assemble wrap

Quick Turkey Wrap

Preparation time: **5 minutes**
Serves 2/Serving size: **1/2 recipe**

2 8-inch flour tortillas
2 Tbsp reduced-fat mayonnaise
1/2 lb sliced turkey breast
1 cup sliced sweet pimientos
1/2 cup sliced dill pickles

1. Place tortillas on the countertop and spread with mayonnaise. Arrange turkey slices on top.
2. Spoon 1/2 cup sweet pimientos on each wrap.
3. Place 1/4 cup dill pickles on each wrap.
4. Roll wrap, slice in half, and serve. If not serving immediately, roll wrap in foil or plastic wrap to keep it from drying out.

Exchanges
2 Starch
4 Very Lean Meat
1 Vegetable
1 1/2 Fat

Calories 392
  Calories from Fat . . 85
Total Fat . . . . 9 g
  Saturated Fat . . . . . . 2 g
Cholesterol . . . . 97 mg
Sodium . . . . 927 mg
Carbohydrate . . . . . 35 g
  Dietary Fiber . . . . . . 4 g
  Sugars . . . . 3 g
Protein . . . . 39 g

Tangerines

Serve 2 tangerines per person.

SHOPPING LIST

STAPLES

Produce
4 tangerines

Deli
1/2 lb sliced turkey breast

Grocery
1 small jar sliced sweet pimientos
1 jar sliced dill pickles
1 package 8-inch flour tortillas

Reduced-fat mayonnaise

chicken wrap

Chicken Avocado Wrap
Oranges

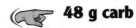 **48 g carb**

Ripe avocado mixed with tomatoes, onion, and hot pepper
sauce makes a tasty, quick filling for colorful tortilla wraps.

HELPFUL HINTS

▌ Some supermarkets carry flavored, colorful
tortillas—look for them!
▌ To help avocados ripen, remove the stem and
place them in a bag in a warm spot.
▌ Choose plain roasted chicken strips or pieces
instead of honey baked, barbecued, or flavored
with sugary coatings.
▌ Using frozen chopped onion is a great
timesaver—keep a bag on hand.

COUNTDOWN

▌ Make filling
▌ Assemble wrap

Chicken Avocado Wrap

Preparation time: **10 minutes**
Serves 2/Serving size: **1/2 recipe**

1/4 peeled onion or 2 Tbsp frozen chopped onion
  1 medium tomato, quartered (about 3/4 cup)
1/2 ripe avocado, peeled and seed removed (about 1/2 cup)
1/2 Tbsp lemon or lime juice
     Several drops hot pepper sauce
     Salt and freshly ground black pepper to taste
  2 8-inch flour tortillas
  2 Tbsp pine nuts
  6 oz roasted boneless skinless chicken breast, cut into strips about
     2 inches long and 1/4 inch wide, or roasted ready-to-eat chicken
     strips (1 1/2 cups)

1. Chop fresh onion in a food processor or add frozen onion, if using. Add tomato, avocado, lemon juice, hot pepper sauce, salt, and pepper. Process to coarsely chop, leaving chunks of avocado.
2. Spread mixture on the two tortillas and sprinkle pine nuts and chicken pieces on top.
3. Roll up each tortilla, cut in half, and serve.

Exchanges
2 Starch
3 Very Lean Meat
1 Vegetable
3 Fat

Calories 423
  Calories from Fat . 146
Total Fat. . . . . 16 g
  Saturated Fat. . . . . . 4 g
Cholesterol. . . . . . 72 mg
Sodium. . . . . 309 mg
Carbohydrate. . . . . 35 g
  Dietary Fiber . . . . . . 5 g
  Sugars. . . . . 4 g
Protein. . . . . 34 g

Oranges

Serve 1 medium orange per person.

SANDWICHES

SHOPPING LIST

Produce
1 small onion
1 small avocado
1 medium tomato
1 lemon or lime
2 medium oranges

Meat
6 oz roasted chicken
  breast

Grocery
1 package 8-inch flour
  tortillas
1 small package pine
  nuts

STAPLES

Hot pepper sauce
Salt
Black peppercorns

egg salad sandwich

**Mediterranean Egg Salad Sandwich
Pears**

 60 g carb

Olives and red peppers are ingredients associated with the
sunny Mediterranean countries. They add zing to this quick egg
salad.

HELPFUL HINTS

▌ You can use already prepared egg salad in
this recipe, but the nutrient analysis may be
different. Add capers and olives in the
amounts below.

▌ You can make egg salad in a food processor.
Be careful to pulse the blades just a few times
to keep it from becoming too finely chopped
or mushy.

▌ Keep hard-boiled eggs in the refrigerator for
snacks or quick salads.

COUNTDOWN

▌ Make hard-boiled
eggs.
▌ While eggs cook,
prepare other
ingredients.
▌ Make egg salad.
▌ Assemble sandwich.

Mediterranean Egg Salad Sandwich

Preparation time: **15 minutes**
Serves 2/Serving size: **1/2 recipe**

6 eggs
2 Tbsp reduced-fat mayonnaise
1 Tbsp Dijon mustard
2 Tbsp water
8 large pitted green olives, coarsely chopped
Salt and freshly ground black pepper to taste
4 slices whole-wheat bread
1 cup sweet pimientos, cut into 2-inch strips

1. Place eggs in a small saucepan and cover with cold water. Place over medium-high heat and bring to a boil. Reduce heat to low and gently simmer 12 minutes.
2. Drain and fill the pan with cold water. When eggs are cool to the touch, peel and cut in half lengthwise. Remove the yolks from 4 of the eggs and discard.
3. Coarsely chop the 6 egg whites and 2 yolks. Set aside.
4. Whisk together mayonnaise, mustard, water, and olives in a bowl. Add eggs and season with salt and pepper. Mix well.
5. Spread the egg salad on four slices of bread. Place pimiento on top. Serve as open-faced sandwiches.

Exchanges
2 Starch
2 Lean Meat
1 Vegetable
1 1/2 Fat

Calories 358
  Calories from Fat . 135
Total Fat. . . . . 15 g
  Saturated Fat. . . . . . 4 g
Cholesterol. . . . . . 218 mg
Sodium. . . . . 1155 mg
Carbohydrate. . . . . 35 g
  Dietary Fiber . . . . . . 6 g
  Sugars. . . . . 6 g
Protein. . . . . 20 g

Pears

Serve 1 medium pear per person.

SHOPPING LIST

Produce
2 medium pears

Dairy
Eggs (6 needed)

Grocery
1 small jar sweet
  pimientos
1 small can or jar pitted
  green olives

STAPLES

Reduced-fat mayonnaise
Dijon mustard
Whole-wheat bread
Salt
Black peppercorns

SANDWICHES

steak sandwich

**Steak and Portobello Mushroom
    Sandwich
Sliced Mango**

 68 g carb

Steak, meaty portobello mushrooms, and sweet onions make a great sandwich. Grill or broil this steak for a leisurely weekend lunch. It tastes best warm or at room temperature.

HELPFUL HINTS

▮ You can use skirt, strip, sirloin, or another quick-cooking steak in this recipe.

▮ If Vidalia onions are not available, use a sweet onion such as Texas Sweet, 1040, or a red onion.

COUNTDOWN

▮ Prepare ingredients
▮ Toast bread
▮ Assemble sandwich

Steak and Portobello Mushroom Sandwich

Preparation time: **15 minutes**
Serves 2/Serving size: **1/2 recipe**

6 oz flank steak
   Salt and freshly ground black pepper to taste
1/4 cup balsamic vinegar
4 medium cloves garlic, crushed
1 cup sliced portobello mushrooms
1 cup sliced Vidalia onion
4 slices whole-wheat bread
   Olive oil cooking spray

1. Remove fat from steak. Heat a nonstick skillet over medium-high heat and add steak. Brown 2 minutes, then turn and brown 2 minutes. Add salt and pepper to the cooked side to keep the meat from losing tasty juices.
2. Mix balsamic vinegar and garlic together.
3. Remove steak to a plate and add mushrooms, onions, and vinegar mixture to the skillet. Sauté 2 minutes.
4. Return steak to skillet for 2 minutes for 1-inch thick steak, 1 minute longer for thicker steak.
5. While steak cooks, spray bread with cooking spray and toast in toaster oven or under a broiler.
6. Slice steak on the diagonal against the grain and divide between 2 slices of bread. Spoon the mushrooms and onions on top. Pour the pan juices over the steak. Add salt and pepper to taste. Cover with 2 remaining slices of bread and cut sandwich in half.

Exchanges
2 Starch
2 Lean Meat
2 Vegetable

Calories 322
  Calories from Fat . . 79
Total Fat . . . . 9 g
  Saturated Fat . . . . . . 3 g
Cholesterol . . . . 40 mg
Sodium . . . . 349 mg
Carbohydrate . . . . . 40 g
  Dietary Fiber . . . . . . 6 g
  Sugars . . . . 12 g
Protein . . . . 24 g

SANDWICHES

Sliced Mango

Serve 1 cup per person.

SHOPPING LIST

Produce
3 oz portobello mushrooms
1 Vidalia onion
1 medium mango

Meat
6 oz flank steak

STAPLES

Garlic
Balsamic vinegar
Olive oil cooking spray
Whole-wheat bread
Salt
Black peppercorns

coleslaw turkey sandwich

**Crunchy Coleslaw
and Turkey Sandwich
Apples**

☞ **49 g carb**

Deli coleslaw with added tomato salsa makes a crunchy topping
for this roast turkey sandwich.

HELPFUL HINTS

▌ Look for deli coleslaw and tomato salsa that
do not have added sugar.
▌ You can use any type of lean deli meat instead
of turkey if you prefer.

COUNTDOWN

▌ Mix coleslaw
▌ Assemble sandwich

Crunchy Coleslaw and Turkey Sandwich

Preparation time: **5 minutes**
Serves 2/Serving size: **1/2 recipe**

1/2 cup prepared or deli coleslaw
  2 Tbsp no-added-sugar tomato salsa
     Salt and freshly ground black pepper to taste
1/2 lb sliced, roasted turkey breast
  4 slices whole-wheat bread

1. Drain coleslaw in a colander.
2. Toss coleslaw with tomato salsa and add salt and pepper.
3. Divide sliced turkey in half and place on 2 slices of bread.
4. Spoon half the coleslaw on top of the turkey and cover with remaining bread slices.
5. Serve extra coleslaw on the side.

Exchanges
2 Starch
4 Very Lean Meat
1 Vegetable
1/2 Fat

Calories 351
   Calories from Fat . . 59
Total Fat. . . . . 7 g
   Saturated Fat. . . . . . 1 g
Cholesterol. . . . . . . 94 mg
Sodium. . . . . 466 mg
Carbohydrate. . . . . 33 g
   Dietary Fiber . . . . . . 5 g
   Sugars. . . . . 8 g
Protein. . . . . 40 g

Apples

Serve 1 small apple per person.

SHOPPING LIST

Produce
2 small apples

Deli
Deli coleslaw
   (3 oz needed)
1/2 lb sliced roasted
   turkey breast

Grocery
1 jar no-added-sugar
   tomato salsa

STAPLES

Whole-wheat bread
Salt
Black peppercorns

roast beef sandwich

Roast Beef Sandwich
   with Tomato and Corn Relish
Fresh Strawberries   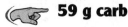 **59 g carb**

This tangy, uncooked relish and roast beef make a tasty, colorful sandwich. Most relishes need slow cooking and lots of sugar. This is a fresh relish and the corn is so sweet that no sugar is needed. It takes very little time to make.

HELPFUL HINT

▌ You can use parsley instead of cilantro if you prefer.

COUNTDOWN

▌ Prepare relish
▌ Assemble sandwich

Roast Beef Sandwich with Tomato and Corn Relish

Preparation time: **10 minutes**
Serves 2/Serving size: **1/2 recipe**

1 cup frozen corn kernels
1 cup diced tomatoes
1 Tbsp balsamic vinegar
2 Tbsp chopped red onion
3 Tbsp fresh cilantro
   Salt and freshly ground black pepper to taste
4 slices whole-wheat bread
6 oz sliced lean roast beef

1. Microwave corn 30 seconds to defrost or place in boiling water for 30 seconds and drain. Mix corn with tomatoes, vinegar, onion, and cilantro. Add salt and pepper.
2. Set relish aside to marinate for a few minutes.
3. Toast bread and place roast beef on 2 slices.
4. Spoon relish over roast beef and cover with remaining slices of bread.

Exchanges
2 1/2 Starch
2 Lean Meat
1 Vegetable

Calories 366
  Calories from Fat . . 62
Total Fat. . . . . 7 g
  Saturated Fat. . . . . . 2 g
Cholesterol. . . . . . . 54 mg
Sodium. . . . . 698 mg
Carbohydrate. . . . . 48 g
  Dietary Fiber . . . . . . 7 g
  Sugars. . . . . 8 g
Protein. . . . . 31 g

Fresh Strawberries

Serve 1 cup per person.

SHOPPING LIST

Produce
1 medium tomato
1 small red onion
1 small bunch cilantro
1 pint strawberries

Deli
6 oz sliced lean roast
  beef

Grocery
1 small package frozen
  corn kernels

STAPLES

Balsamic vinegar
Whole-wheat bread
Salt
Black peppercorns

neapolitan pizza

**Neapolitan Pizza
Plums**

 47 g carb

Neapolitans keep their pizzas simple and tasty. This pizza is topped with fresh tomatoes, a sprinkling of garlic, Parmesan cheese, thinly sliced ham, and a touch of arugula.

HELPFUL HINT

▌ Buy good-quality Parmesan cheese and ask the market to grate it for you or chop it in the food processor. Freeze extra for quick use. You can spoon out the quantity you need and leave the rest frozen.

COUNTDOWN

▌ Preheat broiler
▌ Prepare ingredients
▌ Make pizza

Neapolitan Pizza

Preparation time: **10 minutes**
Serves 2/Serving size: **1/2 recipe**

2 whole-wheat pita breads
2 medium tomatoes, diced (about 2 cups)
2 cloves garlic, crushed
2 tsp olive oil
 Salt and freshly ground black pepper to taste
2 Tbsp grated Parmesan cheese
6 oz lean ham, cut into 2-inch pieces (1 1/4 cups)
1/2 cup torn arugula leaves

1. Preheat broiler and line a baking sheet with foil.
2. Place pita breads on sheet and sprinkle with tomatoes, garlic, and olive oil. Add salt and pepper and sprinkle with Parmesan cheese.
3. Place under broiler 3 minutes. Add ham and return to broiler for 2 minutes.
4. Remove from boiler, sprinkle arugula on top, and serve.

Exchanges
2 Starch
3 Lean Meat
1 Vegetable
1/2 Fat

Calories 373
  Calories from Fat . 117
Total Fat. . . . . 13 g
  Saturated Fat. . . . . . 3 g
Cholesterol. . . . . . 53 mg
Sodium. . . . . . . 1319 mg
Carbohydrate. . . . . 38 g
  Dietary Fiber . . . . . . 4 g
  Sugars. . . . . 7 g
Protein. . . . . 31 g

Plums

Serve 1 medium plum per person.

SHOPPING LIST

Produce
2 medium tomatoes
1 bunch arugula
2 medium plums

Deli
2 oz lean ham

Grocery
1 package whole-wheat pita bread

STAPLES

Parmesan cheese
Garlic
Olive oil
Salt
Black peppercorns

turkey enchiladas

Turkey and Goat Cheese Enchiladas
Fruit-Flavored Yogurt

☞ **44 g carb**

Sliced turkey and tangy goat cheese rolled in a tortilla and topped with a spicy tomato sauce make a quick and satisfying lunch. You can put this enchilada together the night before and warm it up at work the next day.

HELPFUL HINTS

▌ Look for tomato sauce without added sugar or oil. You can use any type of pasta or marinara sauce in this recipe.
▌ If you do not have a microwave, place enchiladas in a toaster oven or under a broiler for 5 minutes.
▌ You can use shredded reduced-fat Mexican cheese instead of Monterey Jack if you wish.

COUNTDOWN

▌ Prepare enchiladas

Turkey and Goat Cheese Enchiladas

Preparation time: **5 minutes**
Serves 2/Serving size: **1/2 recipe**

2 6-inch corn tortillas
1/4 lb sliced turkey breast (scant 1 cup)
2 oz herbed goat cheese (1/3 cup)
1 cup tomato sauce
1/8 tsp hot pepper sauce
2 Tbsp shredded reduced-fat Monterey Jack cheese

1. Place tortillas on the countertop. Divide turkey slices in half and place on each tortilla. Divide goat cheese in half and place on turkey slices.
2. Roll up tortillas and place in a microwave-safe dish just big enough to hold them, seam side down.
3. Mix tomato sauce and hot pepper sauce together and spoon over tortillas.
4. Cover with another dish or plastic wrap and microwave on high for 2 minutes. Remove cover and sprinkle with cheese. Cover and microwave 1 minute.

Exchanges

1 Starch
2 Medium-Fat Meat
1 Vegetable

Calories 251
  Calories from Fat . . 88
Total Fat. . . . . 10 g
  Saturated Fat. . . . . . 6 g
Cholesterol. . . . . . 59 mg
Sodium. . . . . 1450 mg
Carbohydrate. . . . . 21 g
  Dietary Fiber . . . . . . 3 g
  Sugars. . . . . 6 g
Protein. . . . . 23 g

Fruit-Flavored Yogurt

Serve 1 8-oz carton fat-free artificially sweetened fruit-flavored yogurt per person.

SHOPPING LIST

Dairy
2 oz herbed goat cheese
1 small package shredded reduced-fat Monterey Jack cheese
2 8-oz cartons fat-free artificially sweetened fruit-flavored yogurt

Deli
1/4 lb sliced turkey breast

Grocery
1 can or jar tomato sauce
1 package 6-inch corn tortillas

STAPLES

Hot pepper sauce

pita pocket

Greek Tuna Salad Pita Pocket
Cantaloupe

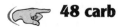 **48 carb**

Feta cheese, olives, cucumbers, and fresh greens are the
base of a typical Greek salad. Add some tuna and serve in a
pita pocket for a quick Greek-style lunch.

HELPFUL HINTS

▌ Feta cheese is sheep's milk cheese and can be
found in the dairy section of the supermarket.
▌ If you don't have pita bread, serve the salad
over 2 slices toasted whole-wheat bread as an
open-faced sandwich.
▌ You can use any type of lettuce.

COUNTDOWN

▌ Prepare ingredients
▌ Assemble sandwich

Greek Tuna Salad Pita Pocket

Preparation time: **5 minutes**
Serves 2/Serving size: **1/2 recipe**

1 cup washed ready-to-eat Romaine lettuce
1 cup cucumber pieces (1/2 inch)
1/2 cup tomato pieces (1/2 inch)
6 oz canned white meat tuna packed in water, drained and flaked
(scant 1 cup drained)
8 pitted black olives, cut in half
2 Tbsp Paul Newman's Oil and Vinegar Salad Dressing
2 whole-wheat pita breads
1 oz crumbled feta cheese (2 Tbsp)

1. Place lettuce, cucumber, tomato, tuna, and olives in bowl and toss with dressing.
2. Cut pita bread in half and open pockets. Fill pockets with salad.
3. Sprinkle feta cheese on top.

Exchanges
2 Starch
3 Lean Meat
1 Vegetable
1 Fat

Calories 382
  Calories from Fat . 135
Total Fat. . . . . 15 g
  Saturated Fat. . . . . . 3 g
Cholesterol. . . . . . . 34 mg
Sodium. . . . . 781 mg
Carbohydrate. . . . . 36 g
  Dietary Fiber . . . . . . 4 g
  Sugars. . . . . 6 g
Protein. . . . . 28 g

Cantaloupe

Serve 1/4 medium cantaloupe per person.

SHOPPING LIST

Produce
1 bag washed ready-to-eat Romaine lettuce
1 cucumber
1 small tomato
1 medium cantaloupe

Dairy
1 package crumbled feta cheese

Grocery
1 small can white meat tuna packed in water
1 can or jar pitted black olives
1 package whole-wheat pita bread

STAPLES

Paul Newman's Oil and Vinegar Salad Dressing

chickpea soup

**Horace's Chickpea Soup
Apples**

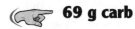 **69 g carb**

La Minestra di Orazio, or Horace's Chickpea and Pasta Soup, is an ancient Roman dish. In one of his satires, Horace is quoted as saying, "I am going home to a bowl of leeks, chickpeas and lasagne. . . ." In fact, this is one of the earliest references to pasta of any kind.

HELPFUL HINTS

▌ Wash leeks by cutting them in half lengthwise, then cutting each half lengthwise again and running them under cold water.
▌ Slice vegetables in a food processor fitted with a slicing blade.

COUNTDOWN

▌ Make soup

Horace's Chickpea Soup

Preparation time: **20 minutes**
Serves 2/Serving size: **1/2 recipe**

- **1** Tbsp olive oil
- **2** medium stalks celery, sliced (1 cup)
- **1** medium leek, sliced (1 cup)
- **2** cups chopped tomatoes
- **1/3** cup acini pepe or orzo pasta
- **3/4** cup canned chickpeas (garbanzo beans), rinsed and drained
- **1 1/2** cups fat-free reduced-sodium chicken broth
- **1/2** cup water
- **1/4** lb lean ham cut into bite-sized pieces (about 1 cup)
  Salt and freshly ground black pepper to taste
- **2** Tbsp freshly grated Parmesan cheese

1. Heat olive oil in a large saucepan over medium-high heat. Add celery and leeks and sauté 3 minutes.
2. Lower heat to medium and add tomatoes. Cook, covered, 5 minutes.
3. Raise heat to high and add pasta, chickpeas, chicken broth, and water. Bring to a boil and cook 8 minutes, stirring occasionally.
4. Stir in ham and add salt and pepper.
5. Serve in large soup bowls with Parmesan cheese sprinkled on top.

Exchanges
2 1/2 Starch
2 Lean Meat
3 Vegetable
1 1/2 Fat

Calories 453
  Calories from Fat . 131
Total Fat. . . . . 15 g
  Saturated Fat. . . . . . 3 g
Cholesterol. . . . . . 37 mg
Sodium. . . . . . . 1337 mg
Carbohydrate. . . . . 53 g
  Dietary Fiber . . . . . . 9 g
  Sugars. . . . . 11 g
Protein. . . . . 30 g

Apples

Serve 1 small apple per person.

SHOPPING LIST

Produce
1 small bunch celery
1 leek
2 medium tomatoes
2 small apples

Deli
1/4 lb lean ham

Grocery
1 can chickpeas
  (garbanzo beans)
1 small package acini
  pepe or orzo pasta

STAPLES

Pamesan cheese
Olive oil
Fat-free reduced-sodium
  chicken broth
Salt
Black peppercorns

tortellini soup

Sausage and Tortellini Soup
Grapefruit

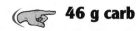 **46 g carb**

Mushroom tortellini and turkey are the base for this quick lunch soup.

HELPFUL HINT

▌ You can use any type of low-fat turkey sausage and fresh or frozen mushroom tortellini in this recipe.

COUNTDOWN

▌ Prepare soup
▌ Prepare fruit

Sausage and Tortellini Soup

Preparation time: **20 minutes**
Serves 2/Serving size: **1/2 recipe**

2 tsp olive oil
1/2 lb low-fat turkey sausage, cut into 1-inch slices
1 cup frozen chopped onions
2 cloves garlic, crushed
2 cups canned diced tomatoes, no added sugar or salt, drained
1 cup fat-free reduced-sodium chicken broth
1 cup water
1/3 cup mushroom tortellini
1 cup basil leaves
    Salt and freshly ground pepper to taste

1. Heat oil in a large nonstick saucepan over medium heat. Add sausage, onion, and garlic and sauté 5 minutes.
2. Add tomatoes, chicken broth, water, and tortellini. Bring to a low boil and cook 5 minutes or until tortellini is cooked through.
3. Remove from heat and stir in basil. Add salt and pepper.

Exchanges
1/2 Starch
2 Lean Meat
5 Vegetable
2 Fat

Calories 368
  Calories from Fat . 144
Total Fat. . . . . 16 g
  Saturated Fat. . . . . . 4 g
Cholesterol. . . . . . . 77 mg
Sodium. . . . . . . 2110 mg
Carbohydrate. . . . . 33 g
  Dietary Fiber . . . . . . 7 g
  Sugars. . . . . 19 g
Protein. . . . . 23 g

Grapefruit

Serve 1/2 large grapefruit per person.

SHOPPING LIST

Produce
1 small bunch fresh basil
1 large grapefruit

Meat
1/2 lb low-fat turkey sausage

Grocery
1 can diced tomatoes, no added sugar or salt
1 cup fat-free reduced-sodium chicken broth
1 small package mushroom tortellini
1 package frozen chopped onions

STAPLES

Olive oil
Garlic
Salt
Black peppercorns

turkey soup

**Turkey and Vegetable Soup
  with Cheddar Bruschetta**
Sliced Mango   **59 g carb**

Quickly slice some vegetables, dice some leftover turkey, and
you can have homemade soup in less than 20 minutes. Double
the recipe and freeze the rest for another delicious meal.

HELPFUL HINTS

▌ Use roasted turkey from the deli.
▌ Use peeled baby carrots to save time.
▌ Most ready-to-eat spinach comes in
   10 oz bags. Just use half a bag for this
   recipe.
▌ Cut French bread on the diagonal to
   make long oval slices.

COUNTDOWN

▌ Prepare soup
▌ Slice fruit
▌ Make bruschetta

Turkey and Vegetable Soup
with Cheddar Bruschetta

Preparation time: **15 minutes**
Serves 2/Serving size: **1/2 recipe**

2 tsp olive oil, divided
1 cup sliced onion
1 cup sliced carrots
2 cups broccoli florets
1 1/2 cups fat-free reduced-sodium chicken broth
1 1/2 cups water
   5 oz washed ready-to-eat spinach (about 5 cups)
   6 oz roasted turkey cut into 1/2- to 1-inch pieces (about 1 cup)
       Salt and freshly ground black pepper to taste
   1 oz shredded reduced-fat cheddar cheese (scant 1/4 cup)
   2 slices whole-grain French bread

1. Heat oil in a large nonstick saucepan over medium-high heat and add onion, carrots, and broccoli. Sauté 5 minutes.
2. Add chicken broth and water. Raise heat, bring to a boil, and cook 5 minutes.
3. Lower heat to medium and add spinach and turkey. Simmer 2 minutes or until turkey is warmed through and spinach is wilted.
4. Add salt and pepper.
5. Sprinkle cheddar cheese on bread slices and toast in toaster oven or under a broiler. Serve with soup.

Exchanges
1 Starch
4 Very Lean Meat
3 Vegetable
1 1/2 Fat

Calories 361
Calories from Fat . . 89
Total Fat. . . . . 10 g
Saturated Fat. . . . . . 3 g
Cholesterol. . . . . . . 79 mg
Sodium. . . . . 777 mg
Carbohydrate. . . . . 31 g
Dietary Fiber . . . . . . 8 g
Sugars. . . . . 11 g
Protein. . . . . 38 g

Sliced Mango

Serve 1 cup mango per person.

SHOPPING LIST

Produce
1 small package peeled baby carrots
1 small package broccoli florets
1 bag washed ready-to-eat spinach
1 large mango

Meat
6 oz roasted turkey

Grocery
1 loaf whole-grain French bread

Dairy
1 small package shredded reduced-fat cheddar cheese

STAPLES

Onion
Olive oil
Fat-free reduced-sodium chicken broth
Salt
Black peppercorns

bean soup

Pasta and Bean Soup
  (Pasta e Fagioli)
Honeydew Melon Cubes

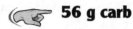 **56 g carb**

The addition of ham to this traditional Italian Pasta and Bean
(Pasta e Fagioli) soup makes it hearty and perfect for lunch.
You can make this 20-minute soup the night before and warm
it up the next day or freeze it for later. You'll want to cook and
add the pasta just before you plan to serve the soup so the pasta
doesn't get mushy.

HELPFUL HINTS

▌ You can use any type of small pasta in this
  soup. It's a good way to use up small quantities of pasta. They can be different shapes
  as long as they're roughly the same size.
▌ If soup is too thick, add more water.
▌ To quickly chop fresh basil, wash, dry, and snip
  the leaves with scissors right off the stem.
▌ Look for honeydew melon cubes in the
  produce section of most supermarkets.

COUNTDOWN

▌ Make soup

Pasta and Bean Soup (Pasta e Fagioli)

Preparation time: **20 minutes**
Serves 2/Serving size: **1/2 recipe**

  1 cup canned cannellini beans, rinsed and drained
  1 clove garlic, crushed
  1 cup sliced celery
  2 cups canned Italian plum tomatoes, drained
1 1/2 cups fat-free reduced-sodium chicken broth
  1/4 cup uncooked small pasta
  1/4 lb lean ham, torn into bite-sized pieces (about 3/4 cup)
      Several drops hot pepper sauce

4–5 sprigs fresh basil, coarsely chopped
2 tsp olive oil
Salt and freshly ground black pepper to taste
2 Tbsp grated Parmesan cheese

1. Place beans, garlic, celery, and tomatoes in a large pot and add chicken broth. Bring to a boil and cover. Lower heat to medium and simmer for 5 minutes.
2. Add pasta and return to a boil. Boil, uncovered, for 9 minutes or until pasta is cooked, stirring occasionally.
3. Remove from heat and add ham, hot pepper sauce, basil, and olive oil. Stir well.
4. Add salt and pepper.
5. Serve in large soup bowls and sprinkle Parmesan cheese on top.

Exchanges

2 Starch

3 Lean Meat

2 Vegetable

Calories 361
Calories from Fat . . 94
Total Fat. . . . . 10 g
Saturated Fat. . . . . . 3 g
Cholesterol. . . . . . . 37 mg
Sodium. . . . . 1671 mg
Carbohydrate. . . . . 40 g
Dietary Fiber . . . . . . 9 g
Sugars. . . . . 8 g
Protein. . . . . 30 g

Honeydew Melon Cubes

Serve 1 cup melon per person.

SHOPPING LIST

Produce
1 bunch celery
1 small bunch basil
1 container honeydew
    melon cubes

Deli
1/4 lb lean ham

Grocery
1 can cannellini beans
1 can Italian plum
    tomatoes
1 package small pasta

STAPLES

Parmesan cheese
Garlic
Fat-free reduced-sodium
chicken broth
Hot pepper sauce
Olive oil
Salt
Black peppercorns

dinner

chinese chicken

Chinese Chicken with Cashew Nuts
Brown Rice with Broccoli
Litchi Cup

 85 g carb

Stir-fried crisp chicken with cashew nuts is a popular
Chinese dish. It's easy and quick to prepare at home.
Chinese recipes have more ingredients than other recipes
but take only a few minutes to cook. It's worth a little extra
effort for true Chinese flavor without extra carbohydrate.

Toasted sesame oil is available in most supermarkets. Toasting
the sesame seeds gives the oil a deep, nutty, sesame flavor.
Rice vinegar is a mild condiment made from fermented rice.

Brown rice takes about 45 minutes to cook, but there are
several brands of quick-cooking brown rice available.
Their cooking time ranges from 10–30 minutes. I find
the 30-minute rice has more flavor, but any quick-cooking
rice will work for this dinner.

I call for a small amount of dry sherry in the chicken recipe. You
can buy small bottles or splits of sherry at most liquor stores.

HELPFUL HINTS

▍ The secret to crisp, not steamed, stir-
frying is to let the ingredients sit for
about a minute when you add them to
the hot wok before you toss them. This
allows the wok to regain its heat after
the cold ingredients have been added.
▍ You can use white vinegar diluted with
a little water instead of rice vinegar in
this recipe.
▍ For easy stir-frying, place all of the prepared ingredients on a cutting board or
plate in order of use. You won't have to
look at the recipe once you start to cook.
▍ Make sure your wok is very hot before
you add the ingredients.

COUNTDOWN

▍ Prepare dessert
▍ Place water for rice on
to boil
▍ Marinate chicken
▍ Prepare chicken
ingredients
▍ Make rice
▍ Stir-fry chicken

POULTRY

Chinese Chicken with Cashew Nuts

Preparation time: **10 minutes**
Serves 2/Serving size: **1/2 recipe**

1/4 cup lite soy sauce
1/4 cup rice vinegar
1/4 cup dry sherry
2 Tbsp chopped fresh ginger (or 2 tsp ground ginger)
3 medium cloves garlic, crushed
1/2 lb boneless skinless chicken breast, cut into 1/2-inch pieces
2 tsp sesame oil
1 medium red bell pepper, sliced (1 cup)
1 tsp cornstarch
Salt and freshly ground black pepper to taste
1/4 cup unsalted cashew nuts
2 scallions, sliced

1. Mix soy sauce, vinegar, sherry, ginger, and garlic together in a small bowl. Add chicken and marinate while you prepare the other ingredients.
2. Heat a wok or skillet over high heat and add oil.
3. Remove chicken from marinade with a slotted spoon, reserving liquid. Add chicken to wok and stir-fry 2 minutes. Remove to a plate.
4. Add red bell pepper and stir-fry 2 minutes.
5. Mix cornstarch with reserved marinade. Add marinade and chicken to the wok and stir-fry 2 minutes with the peppers.
6. Remove from heat. Add salt and pepper. Sprinkle cashew nuts and scallions on top and serve over rice.

Exchanges
1 1/2 Carbohydrate
4 Very Lean Meat
3 Fat

Calories 371
  Calories from Fat . 143
Total Fat. . . . . 16 g
  Saturated Fat. . . . . . 4 g
Cholesterol. . . . . . 68 mg
Sodium. . . . . . . 1281 mg
Carbohydrate. . . . . 21 g
  Dietary Fiber . . . . . . 2 g
  Sugars. . . . . 11 g
Protein. . . . . 30 g

Brown Rice with Broccoli

Preparation time: **30 minutes**
Serves 2/Serving size: **1/2 recipe**

1 1/3 cups water
1/2 cup quick-cooking 30-minute brown rice
2 cups broccoli florets
1 tsp sesame oil
Salt and freshly ground black pepper to taste

1. Bring water to a boil, add rice, lower to medium heat, cover, and cook 25 minutes.
2. Add broccoli florets, cover, and continue to cook 5 minutes. The water should be evaporated. If not, remove the cover and cook a few minutes further. If the rice becomes dry before it is cooked, add more water.
3. Add oil, salt, and pepper.

Exchanges
2 Starch
1 Vegetable
1/2 Fat

Calories 210
Calories from Fat . . 36
Total Fat. . . . . 4 g
Saturated Fat. . . . . . 1 g
Cholesterol. . . . . 0 mg
Sodium. . . . . 22 mg
Carbohydrate. . . . . 39 g
Dietary Fiber . . . . . . 4 g
Sugars. . . . . 1 g
Protein. . . . . 7 g

Litchi Cup

Combine 1/2 cup canned litchis, drained, with
1/2 medium orange, peeled and cut into segments.
Divide into 2 servings.

SHOPPING LIST

Produce
1 medium red bell pepper
1 bunch scallions
1 small piece fresh ginger (or ground ginger)
1 package broccoli florets
1 medium orange

Meat
1/2 lb boneless skinless chicken breast

Grocery
1 small bottle dry sherry
1 small package unsalted cashew nuts
1 can litchis

STAPLES

Garlic
Quick-cooking 30-minute brown rice
Rice vinegar
Lite soy sauce
Sesame oil
Cornstarch
Salt
Black peppercorns

POULTRY

southwestern chicken

Southwestern Chicken
Tortilla Salad
Spiced Berries

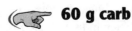 **60 g carb**

Chunky tomato salsa tops sautéed chicken breasts for this 15-minute meal.

HELPFUL HINTS

▌ Flattening the chicken helps it to cook faster. If you skip this step, cook the chicken for 8 instead of 5 minutes after it is browned. A meat thermometer should read 160°F.

▌ Shredded iceberg lettuce and shredded Monterey jack or Mexican-style cheese are available in most supermarkets and only need to be opened and added to this quick salad. Or use another shredded reduced-fat cheese, such as Swiss or cheddar.

▌ Choose bottled salsa without added sugar.

▌ You can use a mixture of berries or one type of berry for dessert.

COUNTDOWN

▌ Make chicken
▌ Assemble salad
▌ Make berries

Southwestern Chicken

Preparation time: **10 minutes**
Serves 2/Serving size: **1/2 recipe**

3/4 lb boneless skinless chicken breast
     Olive oil cooking spray
     Salt and freshly ground black pepper to taste
1 cup bottled chunky no-added-sugar tomato salsa

1. Cut the breasts into 2 6-oz portions and flatten the chicken with the bottom of a heavy skillet or the palm of your hand to about 1/2 inch thick.
2. Heat a medium nonstick skillet over medium-high heat.
3. Spray skillet with cooking spray and add chicken. Brown 2 minutes on each side. Add salt and pepper to the cooked side. Lower heat to medium low and spoon salsa over each chicken portion. Cover and cook 5 minutes.
4. Serve chicken with salsa on top and Tortilla Salad on the side.

Exchanges
5 Very Lean Meat
1 Vegetable
1/2 Fat

Calories 231
  Calories from Fat . . 40
Total Fat. . . . . 4 g
  Saturated Fat. . . . . . 1 g
Cholesterol. . . . . . 103 mg
Sodium. . . . . 426 mg
Carbohydrate. . . . . . 6 g
  Dietary Fiber . . . . . . 1 g
  Sugars. . . . . 3 g
Protein. . . . . 39 g

Tortilla Salad

Preparation time: **5 minutes**
Serves 2/Serving size: **1/2 recipe**

4 cups washed ready-to-eat shredded iceberg lettuce
1 cup canned black beans, rinsed and drained
2 Tbsp shredded reduced-fat Monterey Jack cheese
2 Tbsp Paul Newman's Oil and Vinegar Salad Dressing
1 cup broken tortilla chips

1. Toss iceberg lettuce, black beans, and cheese together in a salad bowl.
2. Add dressing and toss to mix.
3. Sprinkle tortilla chips on top.

Exchanges
2 1/2 Starch
1 Lean Meat
2 Fat

Calories 323
  Calories from Fat . 136
Total Fat. . . . . 15 g
  Saturated Fat. . . . . . 3 g
Cholesterol. . . . . 5 mg
Sodium. . . . . 356 mg
Carbohydrate. . . . . 36 g
  Dietary Fiber . . . . . 10 g
  Sugars. . . . . 4 g
Protein. . . . . 12 g

POULTRY

Spiced Berries

Preparation time: **5 minutes**
Serves 2/Serving size: **1/2 recipe**

1 1/2 cups mixed berries (strawberries, blueberries, or raspberries)
1/4 cup balsamic vinegar
Sugar substitute equivalent to 2 tsp

1. Wash berries and divide between 2 small dessert bowls.
2. Heat balsamic vinegar on high heat for 1 minute or until reduced by one-quarter.
3. Add sugar substitute and stir to dissolve.
4. Pour sauce over berries.

Exchanges
1 Fruit

Calories 70
Calories from Fat . . . 4
Total Fat. . . . . 0 g
Saturated Fat. . . . . . 0 g
Cholesterol. . . . . 0 mg
Sodium. . . . . 4 mg
Carbohydrate. . . . . 18 g
Dietary Fiber . . . . . . 3 g
Sugars. . . . . 11 g
Protein. . . . . 1 g

SHOPPING LIST

Produce
1 package washed shredded ready-to-eat lettuce
1 small package blueberries
1 small package strawberries

Dairy
1 package shredded reduced-fat Monterey Jack cheese

Meat
3/4 lb boneless skinless chicken breast

Grocery
1 small jar chunky no-added-sugar tomato salsa
1 can black beans
1 bag tortilla chips

STAPLES

Olive oil cooking spray
Paul Newman's Oil and Vinegar Salad Dressing
Balsamic vinegar
Sugar substitute
Salt
Black peppercorns

hungarian goulash

Hungarian Goulash
Marinated Mushroom Salad
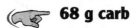 **68 g carb**

A hearty bowl of soup is welcoming at any time of year. Goulash is a traditional Hungarian dish made with bacon, meat, Hungarian paprika, potatoes, and spices.

The secret to this quick soup is Hungarian paprika. It lends a sweet peppery flavor to the soup and can be found in the spice section of some supermarkets. Regular paprika will also work well, but be sure your paprika is fresh.

HELPFUL HINTS

▌ If you like a peppery soup, look for hot Hungarian paprika.
▌ You can use any type of lettuce in the mushroom salad.
▌ The soup gains flavor as it sits. Double the recipe and refrigerate or freeze it for another quick dinner.
▌ Use peeled baby carrots to save time.
▌ Slice vegetables in a food processor.

COUNTDOWN

▌ Make soup
▌ Marinate mushrooms
▌ Assemble salad

Hungarian Goulash

Preparation time: **30 minutes**
Serves 2/Serving size: **1/2 recipe**

Olive oil cooking spray
2 cups sliced red onion
3 cloves garlic, crushed
1 cup sliced celery
1 cup sliced carrots
1 Tbsp Hungarian paprika
2 tsp caraway seeds
2 cups canned whole tomatoes, no added sugar or salt
1 cup water
1/4 lb russet or Idaho potatoes, cut into 1-inch pieces (about 1 cup)
3/4 lb smoked turkey breast, cut into 2-inch strips (about 2 1/2 cups)
Salt and freshly ground black pepper to taste
2 medium slices rye bread
2 Tbsp reduced-fat sour cream

1. Spray a large saucepan with cooking spray and place over medium-high heat. Add onion, garlic, celery, and carrots and sauté 5 minutes.
2. Add paprika, caraway seeds, tomatoes, water, and potatoes. Raise heat to high and bring to a boil, breaking up the tomatoes with a spoon. Cover and cook 10 minutes on high heat.
3. Add smoked turkey breast and continue to cook, covered, 5 minutes. Add salt and pepper.
4. Toast bread and serve on the side.
5. Serve soup in large bowls. Top with 1 Tbsp sour cream each.

Exchanges
2 Starch
4 Very Lean Meat
6 Vegetable
1/2 Fat

Calories 478
Calories from Fat . . 51
Total Fat. . . . . 6 g
Saturated Fat. . . . . . 1 g
Cholesterol. . . . . . . 65 mg
Sodium. . . . . 1966 mg
Carbohydrate. . . . . 64 g
Dietary Fiber . . . . . 12 g
Sugars. . . . . 28 g
Protein. . . . . 47 g

Marinated Mushroom Salad

Preparation time: **5 minutes**
Serves 2/Serving size: **1/2 recipe**

2 cups sliced portobello mushrooms
2 Tbsp Paul Newman's Oil and Vinegar Salad Dressing
Several Romaine lettuce leaves
1 tsp dried dill

1. Toss mushrooms in dressing.
2. Wash lettuce leaves and place on serving plate. Spoon mushrooms on top.
3. Sprinkle with dill.

Exchanges
1 Vegetable
1 1/2 Fat

Calories 98
  Calories from Fat . . 75
Total Fat. . . . . 8 g
  Saturated Fat . . . . . . 1 g
Cholesterol. . . . . . . 0 mg
Sodium. . . . . 80 mg
Carbohydrate. . . . . . 4 g
  Dietary Fiber . . . . . . 1 g
  Sugars. . . . . 2 g
Protein. . . . . 2 g

SHOPPING LIST

Produce
1/4 lb portobello
  mushrooms
1 head Romaine lettuce
1 red onion
1 bunch celery
1 bunch carrots
1/4 lb russet or Idaho
  potatoes

Dairy
1 small carton reduced-
  fat sour cream

Meat
3/4 lb smoked turkey
  breast

Grocery
1 small bottle caraway
  seeds
1 bottle Hungarian
  paprika
1 bottle dried dill
16 oz canned whole
  tomatoes, no added
  sugar or salt

STAPLES

Garlic
Paul Newman's Oil
  and Vinegar Salad
  Dressing
Olive oil cooking spray
Salt
Black peppercorns

POULTRY

chicken cacciatore

Chicken with Green Peppers and
    Tomatoes (Pollo alla Cacciatore)
Linguine   ☜ **69 g carb**

When I first made this classic dish, I asked an Italian friend how to make it. "Don't use red wine; it spoils the dish. Use white wine only," was her emphatic answer. This recipe is a quick 30-minute version of a dish that usually cooks for hours.

The recipe calls for chicken breasts on the bone. Many markets sell them with the wings and skin removed. This will save you a few extra minutes in your kitchen.

HELPFUL HINTS

▌ You can use any shape whole-wheat pasta.
▌ Use peeled baby carrots to save time.
▌ Slice vegetables in a food processor. Slice mushrooms and remove. Then slice carrots, celery, green pepper, and onion together. This way you will not have to wash the bowl in between.

COUNTDOWN

▌ Place water for pasta on to boil
▌ Make chicken
▌ Cook pasta

Chicken with Green Peppers and Tomatoes (Pollo alla Cacciatore)

Preparation time: **20 minutes**
Serves 2/Serving size: **1/2 recipe**

2 8-oz chicken breasts on the bone, skin, wings, and fat removed
1 tsp olive oil
  Salt and freshly ground black pepper to taste
1/2 cup extra dry vermouth
1/2 small onion, sliced (1/2 cup)
  1 medium carrot, thinly sliced (1/2 cup)
  2 medium cloves garlic, crushed
1/2 green pepper, sliced (1/2 cup)
  1 cup sliced portobello mushrooms
  2 cups no-added-salt tomato or marinara sauce
  2 Tbsp grated Parmesan cheese

1. Heat oil in a medium nonstick skillet over medium-high heat. Brown chicken 2 1/2 minutes per side. Add salt and pepper to cooked side.
2. Remove chicken and pour vermouth into skillet, scraping up all of the brown bits.
3. Add onion and carrot. Cover and simmer for 3 minutes. Lower to medium heat.
4. Add garlic, green pepper, mushrooms, and tomato sauce. Return chicken to skillet and gently simmer, covered, for 5 minutes, or until chicken is cooked through. A meat thermometer should read 180°F.
5. Add salt and pepper.
6. Sprinkle Parmesan cheese on top and serve over linguine.

Exchanges
5 Very Lean Meat
5 Vegetable
1 1/2 Fat

Calories	399
Calories from Fat	79
Total Fat	9 g
Saturated Fat	3 g
Cholesterol	117 mg
Sodium	230 mg
Carbohydrate	27 g
Dietary Fiber	5 g
Sugars	21 g
Protein	46 g

POULTRY

Linguine

Preparation time: **10 minutes**
Serves 2/Serving size: **1/2 recipe**

1/4 lb whole-wheat linguine
1 tsp olive oil
Salt and freshly ground black pepper to taste

1. Bring a saucepan with 3–4 quarts water to a boil. Add linguine and boil 9 minutes or according to package instructions.
2. Remove 1/4 cup water from the saucepan and drain linguine. Return linguine to empty pan. Mix olive oil with reserved water and pour over linguine. Toss well.
3. Add salt and pepper.
4. Spoon linguine onto individual plates and serve chicken and sauce over the top.

Exchanges
3 Starch

Calories 230
Calories from Fat . . 35
Total Fat . . . . 4 g
Saturated Fat . . . . . . 0 g
Cholesterol . . . . 0 mg
Sodium . . . . 5 mg
Carbohydrate . . . . . 42 g
Dietary Fiber . . . . . . 3 g
Sugars . . . . 2 g
Protein . . . . 7 g

SHOPPING LIST

Produce
1 medium green pepper
2–3 medium portobello
mushrooms
1 package carrots

Meat
2 8-oz chicken breasts
with bones

Grocery
1 jar or can no-added-salt
tomato or marinara
sauce
1/4 lb fresh or dried
linguine
1 small bottle extra dry
vermouth

STAPLES

Parmesan Cheese
Onion
Garlic
Olive oil
Salt
Black peppercorns

meat loaf

Mediterranean Meat Loaf
Garlic-Whipped Potatoes
Mocha Slush **65 g carb**

Meat loaf in 20 minutes! Here is a modern variation of one of America's favorite comfort foods.

Be sure to look for ground turkey **breast** in the meat section of the supermarket. Unless it is labeled this way, ground turkey may contain fat and skin.

HELPFUL HINTS

▌ Chop all the ingredients for the meat loaf in a food processor.
▌ The coffee slush tastes best when made at the last minute. Since it takes only minutes to make, prepare it after the main course is finished.

COUNTDOWN

▌ Preheat oven to 450°F.
▌ Make meat loaf
▌ Make potatoes
▌ Make meat loaf topping
▌ Make coffee slush just before serving

Mediterranean Meat Loaf

Preparation time: **25 minutes**
Serves 2/Serving size: **1/2 recipe**

1 cup coarsely chopped carrots
1 cup coarsely chopped red onion
1/4 cup plain bread crumbs
3/4 lb ground turkey breast
1 egg white
  Salt and freshly ground black pepper to taste
8 pitted black olives (kalamata if possible), sliced
1/8 tsp crushed red pepper flakes
1 cup canned crushed tomatoes

POULTRY

(Continued)

1. Preheat oven to 450°F.
2. Microwave carrots and onion on high for 3 minutes. They should be slightly shriveled. Mix vegetables with bread crumbs, ground turkey, and egg white. Add salt and pepper. Place a small marble-size piece of the mixture on a plate and microwave 20 seconds. Taste and add more seasoning, if needed.
3. Line a baking sheet with foil. Shape turkey mixture into 2 6 × 3-inch loaves. Bake 15 minutes.
4. Meanwhile, mix olives, pepper flakes, and tomatoes together and microwave on high for 2 minutes or until warmed through.
5. Remove meat loaf from oven and serve with tomato mixture on top.

Exchanges
1/2 Starch
5 Very Lean Meat
5 Vegetable
1/2 Fat

Calories 378
  Calories from Fat . . 37
Total Fat . . . . 4 g
  Saturated Fat . . . . . . 0 g
Cholesterol . . . . . . 105 mg
Sodium . . . . 743 mg
Carbohydrate . . . . . 34 g
  Dietary Fiber . . . . . . 7 g
  Sugars . . . . 16 g
Protein . . . . 49 g

Garlic-Whipped Potatoes

Preparation time: **20 minutes**
Serves 2/Serving size: **1/2 recipe**

1/2 lb yellow potatoes
 16 medium cloves garlic, peeled
  5 Tbsp water (cooking water from potatoes)
    Salt and freshly ground black pepper to taste

1. Wash potatoes, do not peel, and cut into 1-inch pieces. Place in a medium saucepan and add cold water to cover. Cover with a lid and bring to a boil; cook 10 minutes.
2. Add garlic cloves and continue to boil, covered, 5 minutes. Remove 5 Tbsp cooking water and drain potatoes and garlic.

Exchanges
2 Starch

Calories 126
  Calories from Fat . . . 1
Total Fat . . . . 0 g
  Saturated Fat . . . . . . 0 g
Cholesterol . . . . 0 mg
Sodium . . . . 12 mg
Carbohydrate . . . . . 30 g
  Dietary Fiber . . . . . . 3 g
  Sugars . . . . 7 g
Protein . . . . 4 g

3. Pass potatoes and garlic through a potato ricer or food mill or mash by hand. Whisk in reserved water. If using a food processor, add water and process only until just blended, about 5 seconds.
4. Add salt and pepper and serve with meat loaf.

Mocha Slush

Preparation time: **5 minutes**
Serves 2/Serving size: **1/2 recipe**

2 cups diet chocolate soda
2 tsp decaffeinated instant coffee granules
   Sugar substitute equivalent to 2 tsp
30 small ice cubes

Blend ingredients until frothy.

Exchanges
Free Food

Calories 6
   Calories from Fat . . . 0
Total Fat. . . . . 0 g
   Saturated Fat. . . . . . 0 g
Cholesterol. . . . . 0 mg
Sodium. . . . . 15 mg
Carbohydrate. . . . . . 1 g
   Dietary Fiber . . . . . . 0 g
   Sugars. . . . . 1 g
Protein. . . . . 0 g

SHOPPING LIST

Produce
1/2 lb yellow potatoes
1 red onion
1 package carrots

Meat
3/4 lb ground turkey breast

Grocery
1 small can pitted black olives (kalamata if possible)
1 jar crushed red pepper flakes
1 can crushed tomatoes
16 oz diet chocolate soda

STAPLES

Garlic (16 cloves needed)
Plain bread crumbs
Instant decaffeinated coffee
Eggs
Sugar substitute
Salt
Black peppercorns

POULTRY

ginger-minted chicken

Ginger-Minted Chicken
Lemon and Carrot Barley
Honey Pecan Peaches

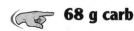 **68 g carb**

If you're in the mood for something different, try this blend of Middle Eastern flavors. Boneless, skinless chicken is marinated in yogurt, spices, mint, and fresh ginger and then broiled. Quick-cooking barley completes the meal. It's flavored with lemon and tossed with shredded carrots that add a crunchy texture to the dish.

HELPFUL HINTS

▌ Quick-cooking barley is available in the grocery section of the supermarket.
▌ Shredded carrots are available in the produce sections of most supermarkets.

COUNTDOWN

▌ Marinate chicken
▌ Preheat broiler
▌ Place water for barley on to boil
▌ Assemble peaches
▌ Cook barley
▌ Broil chicken
▌ Broil peaches

Ginger-Minted Chicken

Preparation time: **35 minutes**
Serves 2/Serving size: **1/2 recipe**

1/2 cup coarsely chopped fresh mint
    1-inch piece fresh ginger, peeled and chopped (about 1 Tbsp, or use 1 tsp ground ginger)
3 medium cloves garlic, crushed
1 cup fat-free plain yogurt
2 tsp ground coriander
2 5-oz. boneless skinless chicken breast halves
1 medium tomato, sliced

1. Mix mint, ginger, and garlic together in a food processor or small bowl. Add yogurt and coriander.

2. Place chicken in a bowl and pour mixture on top. Marinate 15 minutes, turning once during this time.
3. Preheat broiler.
4. Line a baking sheet with foil and place chicken and marinade on sheet.
5. Broil chicken about 5 inches from the heat source for 5 minutes per side.
6. Serve on bed of lemon barley with sliced tomatoes along the side.

Exchanges
4 Very Lean Meat
1 Vegetable
1 Fat-Free Milk

Calories 270
 Calories from Fat . . 35
Total Fat . . . . 4 g
 Saturated Fat . . . . . . 1 g
Cholesterol . . . . . . 88 mg
Sodium . . . . 195 mg
Carbohydrate . . . . . 17 g
 Dietary Fiber . . . . . . 2 g
 Sugars . . . . 13 g
Protein . . . . 40 g

Lemon and Carrot Barley

Preparation time: **15 minutes**
Serves 2/Serving size: **1/2 recipe**

1 1/2 cups water
 1/2 cup quick-cooking barley
   1 cup shredded carrots
   1 Tbsp canola oil
   1 Tbsp chopped fresh thyme (or 1 tsp dried)
   2 Tbsp lemon juice
     Salt and freshly ground black pepper to taste

1. Bring water to a boil and stir in barley. When water returns to a boil, reduce to medium-low heat, partially cover, and simmer 5 minutes. Add carrots, partially cover, and simmer 5 more minutes. If liquid remains, remove cover and boil until it evaporates.
2. Stir oil, thyme, and lemon juice into barley. Add salt and pepper.

Exchanges
2 Starch
1 Vegetable
1 Fat

Calories 215
 Calories from Fat . . 68
Total Fat . . . . 8 g
 Saturated Fat . . . . . . 0 g
Cholesterol . . . . 0 mg
Sodium . . . . 22 mg
Carbohydrate . . . . . 35 g
 Dietary Fiber . . . . . . 6 g
 Sugars . . . . 4 g
Protein . . . . 5 g

POULTRY

Honey Pecan Peaches

Preparation time: **10 minutes**
Serves 2/Serving size: **1/2 recipe**

2 small peaches, pitted and sliced
2 Tbsp pecan pieces
2 tsp honey

1. Preheat broiler.
2. Place peaches in a small shallow baking dish.
3. Drizzle honey over peaches and sprinkle pecans on top. Place under broiler 5 inches from the heat source for 5 minutes.

Exchanges
1 Carbohydrate
1 Fat

Calories	109
Calories from Fat	51
Total Fat	6 g
Saturated Fat	0 g
Cholesterol	0 mg
Sodium	0 mg
Carbohydrate	16 g
Dietary Fiber	2 g
Sugars	13 g
Protein	1 g

SHOPPING LIST

Produce
1 package shredded
   carrots
1 bunch fresh mint
1 bunch fresh thyme or
   1 bottle dried thyme
1-inch piece fresh ginger
   or 1 bottle ground
   ginger
1 medium tomato
1 lemon
2 small ripe peaches

Dairy
1 8-oz carton fat-free
   plain yogurt

Meat
2 5-oz boneless skinless
   chicken breast halves

Grocery
1 package quick-cooking
   barley (in soup section
   of market)
1 bottle ground coriander
1 small package pecan
   pieces

STAPLES

Garlic
Canola oil
Honey
Salt
Black peppercorns

chili

Turkey Chili
Tossed Salad
Sweet Tequila Sunrise 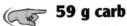 **59 g carb**

This is an intriguing, one-pot turkey chili made the Mexican way—with cinnamon. The turkey marinates for a few minutes in cinnamon with a little vinegar. I first noticed the use of cinnamon in Mexican cooking when I saw a friend add some to the meat she was preparing for her chili. Cinnamon is an East Indian spice that found its way to Mexico through Spain. This is a great way to use leftover turkey or chicken.

HELPFUL HINTS

▌ You can use roasted chicken or turkey.
▌ If you're buying roasted turkey at the deli counter, ask for it to be cut in one 1/2-inch slice weighing about 6 oz.
▌ If you do not have tequila on hand, use any type of liqueur over the orange slices.

COUNTDOWN

▌ Make chili
▌ Assemble salad
▌ Make dessert

POULTRY

Turkey Chili

Preparation time: **25 minutes**
Serves 2/Serving size: **1/2 recipe**

6 oz cooked turkey breast
2 tsp white vinegar
1 tsp ground cinnamon
1 tsp canola oil
1 cup frozen chopped onion
2 medium cloves garlic, crushed
1 cup canned red kidney beans,
   rinsed and drained
2 cups canned whole tomatoes,
   no added sugar or salt
1/2 Tbsp chili powder
1 tsp ground cumin
   Salt and freshly ground
   black pepper to taste
1/2 cup reduced-fat sour cream
1/2 cup fresh chopped cilantro

1. Cut turkey into bite-sized pieces (about 1/2-inch cubes). Place in a bowl and sprinkle with vinegar and cinnamon. Mix well.
2. Heat oil in a medium saucepan over medium-high heat. Add onion and garlic. Sauté about 1–2 minutes. They should not be brown.
3. Add kidney beans, tomatoes, chili powder, and cumin. Break up the tomatoes with a spoon. Simmer gently 15 minutes.
4. Add turkey and simmer 5 more minutes. Add salt and pepper and taste for seasoning. Add more chili powder or cumin as needed.
5. Serve chili with sour cream and cilantro on the side.

Exchanges
2 Starch
4 Very Lean Meat
3 Vegetable
1 Fat

Calories 415
  Calories from Fat . . 87
Total Fat. . . . . 10 g
  Saturated Fat. . . . . . 3 g
Cholesterol. . . . . . . 89 mg
Sodium. . . . . 306 mg
Carbohydrate. . . . . 45 g
  Dietary Fiber . . . . . 11 g
  Sugars. . . . . 16 g
Protein. . . . . 41 g

Tossed Salad

Serve 1 cup washed ready-to-eat salad mix with 1 Tbsp
Paul Newman's Oil and Vinegar Salad Dressing per person.

Sweet Tequila Sunrise

Preparation time: **5 minutes**
Serves 2/Serving size: **1/2 recipe**

1 orange
2 Tbsp tequila
2 Tbsp orange juice

1. Peel orange and slice.
2. Place slices on 2 small dessert plates.
3. Mix tequila and orange juice together and
   spoon over slices.

Exchanges
1 Fruit

Calories 63
  Calories from Fat . . . 1
Total Fat . . . . 0 g
  Saturated Fat . . . . . . 0 g
Cholesterol . . . . 0 mg
Sodium . . . . 0 mg
Carbohydrate . . . . . 11 g
  Dietary Fiber . . . . . . 2 g
  Sugars . . . . 8 g
Protein . . . . 1 g

SHOPPING LIST

Produce
1 bunch cilantro
1 orange
1 bag washed ready-to-
  eat salad mix

Dairy
1 carton reduced-fat
  sour cream
1 small container
  orange juice

Meat
6 oz cooked turkey breast

Grocery
1 can red kidney beans
1 can whole tomatoes,
  no added sugar or salt
1 small bottle tequila
1 package frozen
  chopped onion
1 bottle chili powder
1 bottle ground cumin

STAPLES

Ground cinnamon
White vinegar
Canola oil
Garlic
Paul Newman's Oil
  and Vinegar Salad
  Dressing
Salt
Black peppercorns

POULTRY

meatballs

Middle Eastern Meatballs
Warm Zucchini Salad

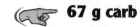 **67 g carb**

The unusual mixture of sweet spices and meat gives a distinctive flavor to Middle Eastern food. You'll love these broiled meatballs placed in warm pita bread pockets to catch the tasty juices. Spoon some freshly chopped parsley, onion, and a little yogurt into the bread to complete this delicious hot sandwich.

HELPFUL HINTS

▌ You can mix the meatball ingredients in a food processor.

COUNTDOWN

▌ Preheat broiler
▌ Make meatballs
▌ Make salad

Middle Eastern Meatballs

Preparation time: **1 minutes**
Serves 2/Serving size: **1/2 recipe**

1/2 lb lean ground round or sirloin
1 cup plus 2 tsp chopped onion, divided
1 egg white
1 tsp ground cinnamon
1/2 tsp salt
2 Tbsp raisins
2 whole-wheat pita breads
1 cup chopped fresh parsley
2 tsp chopped onion
2 Tbsp fat-free plain yogurt

1. Preheat broiler and line a baking sheet with foil.
2. Mix ground beef, 1 cup onion, egg white, ground cinnamon, salt, and raisins together. Blend well. To test for seasoning, take a little bit of the mixture and place on a plate or paper towel, microwave on high 20 seconds, and then taste. Add more cinnamon or salt, if necessary.
3. Roll the mixture into meatballs about 2 inches in diameter and place on a baking sheet.
4. Broil about 5 inches from the heat source for 5 minutes and turn the meatballs over. Broil for another 3–4 minutes. If you like your meatballs more well done, then cook 2–3 minutes longer.
5. While meat is cooking, cut pita breads in half. Place bread on a low rack in the same oven as the meat for 5 minutes to warm through.
6. To serve, open the pita bread pockets and divide the meatballs among them. Sprinkle parsley and onion on top and add 1/2 Tbsp yogurt to each. Serve immediately.

Exchanges
2 Starch
3 Lean Meat
2 Vegetable
1/2 Fruit

Calories 397
  Calories from Fat . . 71
Total Fat. . . . . 8 g
  Saturated Fat. . . . . . 2 g
Cholesterol. . . . . . . 76 mg
Sodium. . . . . 831 mg
Carbohydrate. . . . . 49 g
  Dietary Fiber . . . . . . 5 g
  Sugars. . . . . 15 g
Protein. . . . . 36 g

BEEF

Warm Zucchini Salad

Preparation time: **10 minutes**
Serves 2/Serving size: **1/2 recipe**

1 Tbsp lemon juice
2 cloves garlic, crushed
1 Tbsp olive oil
1/2 cup canned chickpeas (garbanzo beans), rinsed and
    drained
    Salt and freshly ground black pepper to taste
3/4 lb zucchini (about 3 cups)
    Several Romaine lettuce leaves, washed

1. Mix lemon juice and crushed garlic together. Add oil and whisk thoroughly. Add chickpeas, salt, and pepper.
2. Slice zucchini into 1/2-inch rounds. Blanch by bringing a pot half filled with water to a boil and add zucchini. Let water come back to a boil and simmer for 1-2 minutes. Drain and toss in the dressing. Or, microwave on high for 2 minutes and toss with dressing.
3. Serve on a bed of lettuce leaves.

Exchanges
1 Starch
1 Vegetable
1 1/2 Fat

Calories 156
  Calories from Fat . . 67
Total Fat. . . . . 7 g
  Saturated Fat. . . . . . 1 g
Cholesterol. . . . . 0 mg
Sodium. . . . . 69 mg
Carbohydrate. . . . . 18 g
  Dietary Fiber . . . . . . 5 g
  Sugars. . . . . 6 g
Protein. . . . . 6 g

SHOPPING LIST

Produce
1 bunch fresh parsley
2 small zucchini
1 head Romaine lettuce
1 lemon

Dairy
1 8-oz carton fat-free
  plain yogurt

Meat
1/2 lb lean ground round
  or sirloin

Grocery
1 package whole-wheat
  pita bread
1 can chickpeas

STAPLES

Onion
Garlic
Eggs
Raisins
Ground cinnamon
Olive oil
Salt
Black peppercorns

beef kabobs

Honey Mustard Beef Kabobs
Grilled Vegetables
Peach Skewers

 56 g carb

You can make these easy-to-fix kabobs in minutes on an out-door or stove-top grill, or pop them in the broiler. Grilling vegetables gives them a smoky flavor; they can easily be cooked along with the meat.

HELPFUL HINTS

▌ You can use flank, skirt, or another steak suitable for grilling in this recipe.
▌ I call for zucchini and yellow squash, but you can choose a colorful array of whichever vegetables look fresh in the market.
▌ If you broil the kabobs, place them about 2–3 inches from the heat source.
▌ Leave about 1/4 inch between the ingredients on the skewers. This allows the meat and vegetables to cook evenly on all sides.
▌ The peach skewers take only minutes to make. Get them ready to cook, then grill them just before dessert.
▌ Soak wooden skewers in water 10–15 minutes before using them so they don't ignite on the grill.

COUNTDOWN

▌ Preheat grill or broiler
▌ Prepare peach skewers
▌ Prepare vegetables and grill
▌ Prepare beef kabobs and grill
▌ Grill peach skewers

Honey Mustard Beef Kabobs

Preparation time: **10 minutes**
Serves 2/Serving size: **1/2 recipe**

6 Tbsp Dijon mustard
1 Tbsp honey

(Continued)

BEEF

1 tsp Worcestershire sauce
Salt and freshly ground black pepper to taste
3/4 lb boneless sirloin steak, cut into 1-inch cubes

1. Preheat grill or broiler.
2. Combine mustard, honey, and Worcestershire sauce together. Divide mixture, pouring half into 2 small bowls or ramekins to be used as a dipping sauce.
3. Toss beef cubes in remaining sauce, making sure all sides are coated.
4. Thread beef cubes onto skewers and grill or broil 3 minutes. Turn and grill another 3 minutes.
5. Serve with dipping sauce and vegetables.

Exchanges
1 Carbohydrate
4 Lean Meat

Calories 288
Calories from Fat . . 82
Total Fat. . . . . 9 g
Saturated Fat. . . . . . 3 g
Cholesterol. . . . . . . 97 mg
Sodium. . . . . 1187 mg
Carbohydrate. . . . . 14 g
Dietary Fiber . . . . . . 0 g
Sugars. . . . . 14 g
Protein. . . . . 38 g

Grilled Vegetables

Preparation time: **15 minutes**
Serves 2/Serving size: **1/2 recipe**

Olive oil cooking spray
1/2 lb yellow squash (about 2 cups sliced)
1/2 lb zucchini (about 2 cups sliced)
1/2 lb red potatoes (about 2 cups sliced)
2 tsp olive oil
1 medium clove garlic, crushed
1/2 Tbsp water
Salt and freshly ground black pepper to taste

1. Preheat grill or broiler and spray with cooking spray.
2. Wash squash, zucchini, and potatoes. Cut ends off squash and zucchini and cut in half lengthwise. Slice into 1/4-inch strips, yielding 4–5 long strips. Cut potato lengthwise into 1/4-inch slices.
3. Mix olive oil with garlic, water, salt, and pepper together in a medium bowl. Add vegetables and toss to make sure all sides are coated.

Exchanges
1 1/2 Starch
1 Vegetable
1 Fat

Calories 171
Calories from Fat . . 41
Total Fat . . . . 5 g
Saturated Fat. . . . . . 1 g
Cholesterol. . . . . 0 mg
Sodium. . . . . . . 10 mg
Carbohydrate . . . 30 g
Dietary Fiber. . . . . 5 g
Sugars . . . . 6 g
Protein. . . . . 5 g

4. Place vegetables in one layer on grill or broiler pan. Grill or broil 3 minutes, turn vegetables over, and grill or broil 3 minutes more. Remove to a bowl. Cover with foil to keep warm.

Peach Skewers

Preparation time: **10 minutes**
Serves 2/Serving size: **1/2 recipe**

2 medium peaches
1/4 tsp ground allspice
Sugar substitute equivalent to 2 tsp
2 skewers

1. Preheat grill or broiler.
2. Slice peaches in half and remove pit. Cut each half into 3 large slices.
3. Mix allspice and sugar substitute together and toss peach slices in mixture, making sure all of the slices are coated.
4. Place slices on skewers and grill or broil 3 minutes, turn fruit over, and grill or broil 3 minutes more.
5. Serve warm.

Exchanges
1 Fruit

Calories 48
  Calories from Fat . . . 1
Total Fat. . . . . 0 g
  Saturated Fat. . . . . . 0 g
Cholesterol. . . . . 0 mg
Sodium. . . . . 0 mg
Carbohydrate. . . . . 12 g
  Dietary Fiber . . . . . . 2 g
  Sugars. . . . . 10 g
Protein. . . . . 1 g

SHOPPING LIST

Produce
1/2 lb yellow squash
1/2 lb zucchini
1/2 lb red potatoes
2 medium peaches

Meat
3/4 lb boneless sirloin
  steak

Grocery
1 bottle allspice

STAPLES

Olive oil cooking spray
Olive oil
Garlic
Honey
Sugar substitute
Dijon mustard
Worcestershire sauce
Salt
Black peppercorns

BEEF

chinese pepper steak

Chinese Pepper Steak
Quick Stir-Fried Rice
Pineapple Chunks

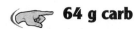 **64 g carb**

You'll be stir-frying thin slices of beef in a savory mixture of green peppers, fresh ginger, and garlic to make this tasty dish. Chinese food takes only minutes to cook; it's the chopping and cutting that take some time. To speed things up, look for pre-sliced beef and stir-fry vegetables in the supermarket. Or slice vegetables in a food processor.

Use the same wok to make the rice—the pan juices from the meat will flavor it. Fried rice is great made with leftover rice.

HELPFUL HINTS

▌ You can use skirt or flank steak instead of sirloin.
▌ You'll need chopped onion for both recipes, so prepare it all at once and divide accordingly.
▌ Your wok or skillet should be very hot when you add the vegetables and meat.

COUNTDOWN

▌ Place water for rice on to boil
▌ Prepare beef ingredients
▌ Boil rice
▌ Stir-fry beef
▌ Stir-fry rice

Chinese Pepper Steak

Preparation time: **10 minutes**
Serves 2/Serving size: **1/2 recipe**

  1 tsp sesame oil
1/2 medium onion, sliced (1 cup)
  2 medium green bell peppers, sliced (about 3 cups)
  1 Tbsp chopped fresh ginger or 1 tsp ground ginger
  3 medium cloves garlic, crushed
1/2 lb sirloin steak, cut into 2 × 1/2-inch strips
  2 Tbsp lite soy sauce

1. Heat sesame oil in wok. When wok is smoking, add
   onion, green pepper, ginger, and garlic. Stir-fry
   3 minutes.
2. Add meat and stir-fry 1 minute.
3. Add soy sauce and stir-fry 3 minutes. Remove to a plate.
   Do not wash wok; use it to stir-fry cooked rice.

Exchanges
3 Lean Meat
3 Vegetable

Calories 242
   Calories from Fat . . 69
Total Fat. . . . . 8 g
   Saturated Fat. . . . . . 2 g
Cholesterol. . . . . . . 64 mg
Sodium. . . . . 661 mg
Carbohydrate. . . . . 19 g
   Dietary Fiber . . . . . . 4 g
   Sugars. . . . . 11 g
Protein. . . . . 25 g

BEEF

Quick Stir-Fried Rice

Preparation time: **15 minutes**
Serves 2/Serving size: **1/2 recipe**

1/2 cup long-grain white rice
  2 tsp sesame oil
1/4 cup sliced onion
    Salt and freshly ground black pepper to taste

1. Bring a large pot with 2–3 quarts of water to
   a boil. Add rice and boil, uncovered, about
   10 minutes. Test a grain. Rice should be cooked
   through but not soft. Drain into a colander in
   the sink.
2. Add oil to wok and heat to smoking. Add onion
   and stir-fry 1 minute. Add rice and stir-fry
   2–3 minutes. Add salt and pepper.

Exchanges
2 1/2 Starch
1/2 Fat

Calories 201
  Calories from Fat . . 44
Total Fat. . . . . 5 g
  Saturated Fat. . . . . . 1 g
Cholesterol. . . . . 0 mg
Sodium. . . . . 2 mg
Carbohydrate. . . . . 35 g
  Dietary Fiber . . . . . . 1 g
  Sugars. . . . . 1 g
Protein. . . . . 3 g

Pineapple Chunks

Serve 1/2 cup per person.

SHOPPING LIST

Produce
2 medium green bell
  peppers
1 small piece fresh ginger
1 package fresh pineapple
  chunks

Meat
1/2 lb sirloin steak

STAPLES

Long-grain white rice
Onion
Garlic
Sesame oil
Lite soy sauce
Salt
Black peppercorns

korean beef

Korean Grilled Beef
Green Rice
Almond-Stuffed Pears

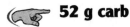 **52 g carb**

Steak plays an important role in Korean cooking, unlike other Asian cuisines. Invading Mongols brought beef to Korea in the Middle Ages. Rice cooked with spinach and bean sprouts is another Korean staple. I have adapted these recipes to showcase the intriguing flavors of Korean cooking while reducing preparation time.

HELPFUL HINTS

- You can use flank, strip, or sirloin instead of skirt steak.
- This beef works well on an outdoor or stove-top grill, or you can broil it.
- Most washed, ready-to-eat spinach is sold in 10 oz bags. Use half a bag for this recipe.

COUNTDOWN

- Marinate beef
- Make pears
- Make rice
- Preheat grill or broiler
- Grill beef

Korean Grilled Beef

Preparation time: **25 minutes**
Serves 2/Serving size: **1/2 recipe**

3/4 lb skirt steak
  2 Tbsp lite soy sauce
  2 Tbsp white vinegar
  2 cloves garlic, crushed
  2 tsp Dijon mustard
    Salt and freshly ground black pepper to taste

1. Score meat deeply crosswise at 1/2-inch intervals. This allows the meat to absorb more of the marinade and cook more evenly.

BEEF

2. Mix soy sauce, vinegar, garlic and mustard together. Add meat and turn in the marinade to make sure all sides are coated with the sauce. Marinate for 10 minutes.
3. Preheat grill or broiler. Remove meat and discard marinade. Place on grill or broiler about 3–4 inches from the heat source. Grill 5–7 minutes. A meat thermometer should read 145 °F. Remove to a carving board and add salt and pepper to the cooked steak.
4. Slice steak across the grain, making sure to capture the juices.
5. Serve over Green Rice, and pour the juices on top.

Exchanges
4 Lean Meat

Calories 220
  Calories from Fat . . 67
Total Fat. . . . . 7 g
  Saturated Fat. . . . . . 3 g
Cholesterol. . . . . . . 97 mg
Sodium. . . . . 557 mg
Carbohydrate. . . . . . 2 g
  Dietary Fiber . . . . . . 0 g
  Sugars. . . . . 2 g
Protein. . . . . 34 g

Green Rice

Preparation time: **35 minutes**
Serves 2/Serving size: **1/2 recipe**

  5 oz washed ready-to-eat fresh spinach
1/2 cup quick-cooking 30-minute brown rice
  1 cup fresh bean sprouts
  1 cup water
  2 tsp sesame oil
  2 scallions, sliced
    Salt and freshly ground black pepper to taste

1. Place spinach, rice, bean sprouts, and water in a large saucepan. Bring the water to a boil and cover with a lid. Lower heat to medium and simmer 30 minutes or according to package instructions. The water should be absorbed and the rice cooked through. If the rice is cooked and there is still liquid in the pan, remove lid and boil to evaporate liquid.
2. Stir in sesame oil and scallions. Add salt and pepper.
3. Place on dinner plate. Serve sliced steak on top.

Exchanges
1 1/2 Starch
1 Vegetable
1 Fat

Calories 171
  Calories from Fat . . 51
Total Fat. . . . . 6 g
  Saturated Fat. . . . . . 1 g
Cholesterol. . . . . 0 mg
Sodium. . . . . 72 mg
Carbohydrate. . . . . 27 g
  Dietary Fiber . . . . . . 4 g
  Sugars. . . . . 2 g
Protein. . . . . 6 g

Almond-Stuffed Pears

Preparation time: **5 minutes**
Serves 2/Serving size: **1/2 recipe**

2 small ripe pears
2 Tbsp slivered almonds
2 tsp almond extract
   Garnish
   Mint leaves (optional)

1. Slice pears in half and remove core. Cut a thin slice from the rounded side of the pear so that it will sit flat.
2. Toast slivered almonds in a toaster oven until slightly golden, about 30 seconds.
3. Place pear halves on 2 small dessert plates and sprinkle almond extract in the cored center of each half.
4. Spoon slivered almonds in the cored center and place sprig of mint on the side.

Exchanges
1 1/2 Fruit
1 Fat

Calories 141
  Calories from Fat . . 42
Total Fat. . . . . 5 g
  Saturated Fat. . . . . . 0 g
Cholesterol. . . . . . . 0 mg
Sodium. . . . . 1 mg
Carbohydrate. . . . . 23 g
  Dietary Fiber . . . . . . 4 g
  Sugars. . . . . 18 g
Protein. . . . . 2 g

SHOPPING LIST

Produce
1 bunch scallions
1 10-oz package washed
   ready-to-eat spinach
1 package fresh bean
   sprouts
2 small ripe pears
1 small bunch fresh
   mint (optional)

Meat
3/4 lb skirt steak

Grocery
1 bottle almond extract
1 small package slivered
   almonds

STAPLES

Garlic
Dijon mustard
White vinegar
Lite soy sauce
Sesame oil
Quick 30-minute
   brown rice
Salt
Black peppercorns

BEEF

picadillo

Picadillo
Tomato and Onion Salad
Cheddar Cheese and Apples   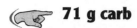 **71 g carb**

Picadillo, or ground meat in a flavor-packed tomato sauce, is a popular Cuban dish served in many Latin restaurants. There are many Picadillo variations, but olives and capers are always part of the recipe. It was served at Sloppy Joe's Bar in Key West over rolls and became known there as Sloppy Joes. On a roll or not, it's a quick and delicious dish that can be made a day ahead or frozen for later.

HELPFUL HINTS

▯ Look for lean ground round or sirloin.
▯ To quickly chop fresh herbs, wash, dry, and snip the leaves with scissors right off the stem.
▯ You'll need chopped onion for both recipes, so prepare it all at once and divide accordingly.
▯ If you are pressed for time, use frozen chopped onion and green pepper.

COUNTDOWN

▯ Make picadillo
▯ Make salad
▯ Assemble dessert

Picadillo

Preparation time: **20 minutes**
Serves 2/Serving size: **1/2 recipe**

1 tsp olive oil	1 Tbsp drained capers
1 cup diced red onion	2 Tbsp Worcestershire sauce
2 cloves garlic, crushed	2 Tbsp white vinegar
1 cup diced green bell pepper	Salt and freshly ground
1/2 lb lean ground round	black pepper to taste
1 1/2 cups canned tomato sauce	2 small whole-wheat rolls

1. Heat oil in a nonstick skillet over medium-high heat. Add onion, garlic, and green pepper. Sauté 5 minutes.
2. Add beef and brown, breaking it up into small pieces as it browns. Drain fat.
3. Add tomato sauce and mix well. Add capers, Worcestershire sauce, and white vinegar. Lower heat to medium and cook at a simmer, stirring occasionally, until meat is cooked through, about 10 minutes.
4. Taste for seasoning. Add salt and pepper and more vinegar and Worcestershire sauce, if necessary.
5. Serve on rolls.

Exchanges
1 Starch
3 Lean Meat
5 Vegetable

Calories 359
  Calories from Fat . . 63
Total Fat . . . . 7 g
  Saturated Fat . . . . . . 2 g
Cholesterol . . . . . . 58 mg
Sodium . . . . 581 mg
Carbohydrate . . . . . 45 g
  Dietary Fiber . . . . . . 6 g
  Sugars . . . . 23 g
Protein . . . . 28 g

Tomato and Onion Salad

Preparation time: **5 minutes**
Serves 2/Serving size: **1/2 recipe**

2 medium tomatoes, sliced
1/4 cup diced red onion
2 Tbsp Paul Newman's Oil and Vinegar Salad Dressing
  Salt and freshly ground black pepper

1. Arrange tomatoes on a serving plate.
2. Sprinkle diced onion on top of tomatoes and drizzle dressing over both.
3. Add salt and pepper.

Exchanges
2 Vegetable
1 1/2 Fat

Calories 114
  Calories from Fat . . 77
Total Fat . . . . 9 g
  Saturated Fat . . . . . . 1 g
Cholesterol . . . . 0 mg
Sodium . . . . 89 mg
Carbohydrate . . . . . . 9 g
  Dietary Fiber . . . . . . 2 g
  Sugars . . . . 6 g
Protein . . . . 1 g

BEEF

Cheddar Cheese and Apples

Preparation time: **5 minutes**
Serves 2/Serving size: **1/2 recipe**

2 small apples
1 Tbsp lemon juice
2 oz reduced-fat sharp Cheddar cheese

1. Core apples and cut into thin slices.
2. Divide slices between 2 small dessert plates.
3. Sprinkle with lemon juice.
4. Cut cheese into strips and serve over slices.

Exchanges
1 Medium-Fat Meat
1 Fruit

Calories 145
  Calories from Fat . . 58
Total Fat. . . . . 6 g
  Saturated Fat. . . . . . 4 g
Cholesterol. . . . . . . 20 mg
Sodium. . . . . 242 mg
Carbohydrate. . . . . 17 g
  Dietary Fiber . . . . . . 3 g
  Sugars. . . . . 14 g
Protein. . . . . 7 g

SHOPPING LIST

Produce
1 red onion
1 medium green bell
  pepper
2 medium tomatoes
1 lemon
2 small apples

Dairy
1 small package reduced-
  fat sharp Cheddar
  cheese

Meat
1/2 lb lean ground round

Grocery
1 can tomato sauce
  (12 oz needed)
1 jar pitted green olives
1 small jar capers

STAPLES

Olive oil
Paul Newman's Oil and
  Vinegar Salad Dressing
Garlic
Worcestershire sauce
White vinegar
Salt
Black peppercorns

veal rolls

Stuffed Veal Rolls
Parmesan Tomatoes and Beans
Strawberry-Banana Cup

 50 g carb

Stuffed Veal rolls is a popular dish in Emilia-Romagna, a rich and fertile area of Northern Italy where veal is a specialty.

HELPFUL HINTS

▌ You can use a good cheddar or Swiss cheese instead of Parmesan.

▌ Buy good-quality Parmesan cheese and ask the market to grate it for you or chop it in the food processor. Freeze extra for quick use. You can spoon out the quantity you need and leave the rest frozen.

▌ You can use any type of canned white beans.

▌ Make sure your veal cutlets are about the same size. If not, cut the bigger pieces to match the smaller ones. They will cook more evenly this way.

▌ You can turn the veal rolls easily with kitchen tongs.

COUNTDOWN

▌ Prepare fruit

▌ Make beans and cover with a lid to keep warm

▌ Make veal

VEAL

Stuffed Veal Rolls

Preparation time: **15 minutes**
Serves 2/Serving size: **1/2 recipe**

3/4 lb thinly cut veal cutlets, fat trimmed
Salt and freshly ground black pepper to taste
1 bunch arugula (1 cup), washed and patted dry
1 bunch basil (1 cup), washed and patted dry
1 tsp olive oil
1/2 cup dry vermouth
1/2 cup fat-free reduced-sodium chicken broth
Wooden toothpicks

1. Spread the veal out on a cutting board or countertop and flatten with a meat mallet or bottom of a heavy skillet to 1/4-inch thick. Salt and pepper the veal pieces.
2. Place a layer of arugula over the veal, making sure the surface is covered. Place a layer of basil leaves over the arugula. Roll up meat and fasten with a wooden toothpick.
3. Heat oil in a nonstick skillet just large enough to hold the veal in one layer. Brown veal rolls on all sides, about 3 minutes. Remove to a dish and cover with foil to keep warm.
4. Add vermouth to the skillet. Let reduce about 2 minutes, scraping up the brown bits as it cooks. Add broth. Let reduce again about 5 minutes. Return veal to the sauce to let it warm through for a minute. If rolls are thick, warm for 3–4 minutes.
5. Remove rolls and slice into 2-inch pieces. Place on plates with the sliced side up so that the colorful interior is shows. Spoon sauce over the top.

Exchanges
4 Lean Meat
1/2 Fat

Calories 256
  Calories from Fat . . 65
Total Fat. . . . . 7 g
  Saturated Fat. . . . . . 2 g
Cholesterol. . . . . . 134 mg
Sodium. . . . . 197 mg
Carbohydrate. . . . . . 2 g
  Dietary Fiber . . . . . . 1 g
  Sugars. . . . . 0 g
Protein. . . . . 38 g

Parmesan Tomatoes and Beans

Preparation time: **10 minutes**
Serves 2/Serving size: **1/2 recipe**

1/2 cup fat-free reduced-sodium chicken broth
1/2 cup canned cannellini beans, rinsed and drained
  2 medium tomatoes, diced (about 2 cups)
  2 Tbsp grated Parmesan cheese
     Salt and freshly ground black pepper to taste

1. Add broth, beans, and tomatoes to a medium saucepan. Bring to a simmer. Cook 5 minutes or until beans and tomatoes are warmed through.
2. Add Parmesan cheese, salt, and pepper. Toss well.

Exchanges
1 Starch
1 Lean Meat

Calories 123
  Calories from Fat . . 24
Total Fat. . . . . 3 g
  Saturated Fat. . . . . . 1 g
Cholesterol. . . . . 5 mg
Sodium. . . . . 231 mg
Carbohydrate. . . . . 19 g
  Dietary Fiber . . . . . . 5 g
  Sugars. . . . . 5 g
Protein. . . . . 8 g

Strawberry-Banana Cup

Serve 1/2 cup sliced fresh strawberries mixed with 1/4 cup sliced bananas per person.

SHOPPING LIST

Produce
1 bunch arugula
1 bunch basil
2 medium tomatoes
1 small container
  strawberries
1 medium banana

Meat
1/2 lb veal cutlets, thinly
  cut

Grocery
1 small bottle dry
  vermouth
1 can cannellini beans

STAPLES

Parmesan cheese
Fat-free reduced-sodium
  chicken broth
Olive oil
Salt
Black peppercorns

VEAL

veal gorgonzola

Veal Gorgonzola
Fresh Linguine and Artichoke Hearts
Frozen Yogurt

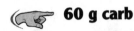 **60 g carb**

Veal with Gorgonzola sauce perfectly blends ingredients from the Lombardy region in northern Italy, which stretches all the way to the Alps. Gorgonzola is a blue-veined, mild cheese that takes its name from a town in Lombardy. You can easily find a domestic Gorgonzola in the supermarket that works very well in this recipe.

HELPFUL HINTS

▌ Look for crumbled, domestic Gorgonzola in the dairy section of the market, or you can use any type of blue veined cheese.
▌ Use a nonstick skillet that just fits the veal in one layer. If your skillet is too big, the sauce will evaporate.
▌ Fresh linquine is best in this recipe, but you can use dried instead.
▌ Marinated artichoke hearts can be found in most supermarkets.

COUNTDOWN

▌ Make salad
▌ Make veal

Veal Gorgonzola

Preparation time: **10 minutes**
Serves 2/Serving size: **1/2 recipe**

1	Tbsp flour
	Salt and freshly ground black pepper to taste
2	4-oz veal cutlets, fat trimmed
	Olive oil cooking spray
1/2	cup fat-free milk
2 1/2	Tbsp crumbled Gorgonzola cheese

1. Place flour on a plate and season with salt and pepper.
2. Dip veal cutlets in the flour, making sure both sides are coated.
3. Heat a small nonstick skillet over medium-high heat and spray with cooking spray. Add one cutlet and brown 2 minutes. Turn and brown 1 minute. Transfer to serving dish and add second cutlet to skillet. Brown 2 minutes, turn, and brown 1 minute. Remove to serving dish and sprinkle both cutlets with salt and pepper.
4. Add milk to the skillet and scrape up the brown bits in the bottom of the pan.
5. Immediately add cheese and stir to melt cheese and make a smooth sauce. Taste for seasoning. Add pepper if needed (the cheese should provide enough salt).
6. Spoon sauce over cutlets and serve.

Exchanges
1/2 Starch
3 Lean Meat

Calories	197
Calories from Fat	57
Total Fat	6 g
Saturated Fat	3 g
Cholesterol	82 mg
Sodium	230 mg
Carbohydrate	6 g
Dietary Fiber	0 g
Sugars	3 g
Protein	27 g

VEAL

Fresh Linguine and Artichoke Hearts

Preparation time: **15 minutes**
Serves 2/Serving size: **1/2 recipe**

1/4 lb fresh spinach linguine
  1 tsp olive oil
3/4 cup drained marinated artichoke hearts, cut into
    small pieces
    Salt and freshly ground black pepper to taste

1. Place a large saucepan with 3–4 quarts water on to boil.
2. Add linguine and boil 3 minutes.
3. Drain, leaving about 2 Tbsp water on pasta.
4. Add oil, artichoke hearts, salt, and pepper. Toss well.

Exchanges
2 Starch
1 Vegetable
1 Fat

Calories 223
  Calories from Fat . . 54
Total Fat. . . . . 6 g
  Saturated Fat. . . . . . 1 g
Cholesterol. . . . . 0 mg
Sodium. . . . . 256 mg
Carbohydrate. . . . . 34 g
  Dietary Fiber . . . . . . 2 g
  Sugars. . . . . 1 g
Protein. . . . . 8 g

Frozen Yogurt

Serve 1/2 cup low-fat frozen yogurt per person.

SHOPPING LIST

Dairy
1 small package
  crumbled Gorgonzola
  cheese (1 oz needed)

Meat
2 4-oz veal cutlets

Grocery
1/4 lb fresh spinach
  linguine
1 jar marinated
  artichokes
1 carton low-fat frozen
  yogurt

STAPLES

Flour
Olive oil
Olive oil cooking spray
Fat-free milk
Salt
Black peppercorns

roasted pork

Mojo Roasted Pork
Cuban Rice and Beans
Pears with Pineapple Sauce   **58 g carb**

Caribbean restaurants have become popular in many cities throughout the States. I have created these flavorful, simple, Cuban-style recipes that you can make at home in minutes.

A garlicky mojo glaze coats this pan-roasted pork tenderloin. Mojo is a Cuban condiment and marinade that is used in many Cuban recipes. There are many versions, but it's usually made with Seville or sour oranges, spices, garlic, onion, and oil. You can find it bottled in most supermarkets, sometimes under the name Spanish barbecue sauce. The bottled version is perfect for this quick pork dinner. Look for one that is low in fat. Some have no fat.

If you can't find mojo in your store, use this quick substitute. It's not very authentic, but it works well for this recipe: mix together 1/4 cup orange juice, 1/4 cup lemon or lime juice, and 3 garlic cloves, crushed; add a little salt and pepper and use as the marinade. (The nutrition analysis for the pork was calculated using this recipe without added salt or pepper.)

HELPFUL HINTS

▎ You can use red beans instead of black.
▎ Look for rum in small splits similar to the size served on airplanes. Or, use an orange-flavored liqueur.
▎ To save time, measure the mojo sauce in a glass liquid measuring cup and marinate the pork in the cup.

COUNTDOWN

▎ Marinate pork
▎ Set water for rice on to boil
▎ Make rice
▎ Make pork
▎ Make dessert

Mojo Roasted Pork

Preparation time: **25 minutes**
Serves 2/Serving size: **1/2 recipe**

(Continued)

PORK

3/4 lb pork tenderloin
1/2 cup mojo sauce
 1 Tbsp low-sugar apricot spread

1. Remove fat from pork and butterfly it by cutting the pork in half lengthwise and opening it like a book. Do not cut all the way through. Place pork in the mojo and let marinate for 15 minutes.
2. Heat a nonstick skillet over medium-high heat. Remove pork, reserving marinade. Pat dry with paper towel and sauté in skillet 3 minutes. Turn and sauté 3 minutes. The pork is done when a meat thermometer reads 160°F.
3. Mix reserved marinade and apricot spread together. Remove pork to a plate and add marinade mixture to the skillet. Boil about 1 minute, scraping up the brown bits in the pan as it boils. Divide pork into 2 portions, place on dinner plates, and spoon sauce over the top.

Exchanges
1/2 Carbohydrate
4 Lean Meat

Calories 241
 Calories from Fat . . 56
Total Fat . . . . 6 g
 Saturated Fat . . . . . . 2 g
Cholesterol . . . . 97 mg
Sodium . . . . 84 mg
Carbohydrate . . . . . 10 g
 Dietary Fiber . . . . . . 0 g
 Sugars . . . . 8 g
Protein . . . . 36 g

Cuban Rice and Beans

Preparation time: **35 minutes**
Serves 2/Serving size: **1/2 recipe**

1/3 cup quick-cooking 30-minute brown rice
1/2 cup sliced onion
 1 cup green bell pepper, sliced
3/4 cup canned black beans, rinsed and drained
 4 tsp canola oil
 Salt and freshly ground black pepper to taste

1. Bring a large saucepan with 2–3 quarts of water to a boil. Add rice and boil rapidly 27 minutes.
2. Add onion and pepper and continue to boil 3 minutes or until the rice is cooked through but still firm.
3. Drain rice mixture and place in a bowl. Add black beans and oil and toss well. Add salt and pepper.

Exchanges
2 Starch
1 Vegetable
2 Fat

Calories 252
 Calories from Fat . . 90
Total Fat . . . . 10 g
 Saturated Fat . . . . . . 1 g
Cholesterol . . . . 0 mg
Sodium . . . . 91 mg
Carbohydrate . . . . . 35 g
 Dietary Fiber . . . . . . 8 g
 Sugars . . . . 5 g
Protein . . . . 8 g

Pears with Pineapple Sauce

Preparation time: **5 minutes**
Serves 2/Serving size: **1/2 recipe**

1 ripe medium pear
1/2 cup fresh pineapple cubes
   Sugar substitute equivalent to 1 tsp
1/2 Tbsp light rum
   Several mint leaves for garnish (optional)

1. Slice pears in half and remove core. Cut a thin slice from the rounded side of the pear so that it will sit flat. Place on 2 dessert plates rounded side down.
2. Purée pineapple, sugar substitute, and rum together in a food processor or blender. Spoon over pears.
3. Place mint leaves on the side for garnish.

Exchanges
1 Fruit

Calories	77
Calories from Fat	4
Total Fat	0 g
Saturated Fat	0 g
Cholesterol	0 mg
Sodium	0 mg
Carbohydrate	18 g
Dietary Fiber	2 g
Sugars	15 g
Protein	0 g

SHOPPING LIST

Produce
1 ripe pear
1 medium green bell pepper
1 small package fresh pineapple cubes
1 small bunch fresh mint (optional)

Meat
3/4 lb pork tenderloin

Grocery
1 small bottle mojo sauce
1 bottle low-sugar apricot spread
1 can black beans
1 small bottle or 1 split light rum

STAPLES

Onion
Canola oil
Quick-cooking 30-minute brown rice
Sugar substitute
Salt
Black peppercorns

PORK

cider pork

Cider Pork
Autumn Squash
Apricot Fool

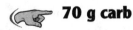 **70 g carb**

When I saw the markets filled with autumn colors and flavors, golden jugs of cider, green and orange squash, and an array of colorful nuts, I was inspired to create this Cider Pork. It's simple to make and I find the apple flavor enhances the pork and rosemary.

HELPFUL HINTS

▌ To save time, wash the squash but do not peel it.
▌ To quickly chop fresh rosemary, wash, dry, and snip the leaves with scissors right off the stem.
▌ You can use frozen uncooked squash or pumpkin cubes. Simply sauté the onions, add the frozen squash, and cook until defrosted.
▌ Sauté the squash and then let it finish cooking in the heat of the pan off the burner. This method allows the squash to develop its delicate texture while you prepare the rest of the meal.

COUNTDOWN

▌ Make squash
▌ Make pork
▌ Make dessert

Cider Pork

Preparation time: **20 minutes**
Serves 2/Serving size: **1/2 recipe**

3/4 lb pork tenderloin
1 Tbsp fresh rosemary (or 2 tsp dried)
2 tsp olive oil
 Salt and freshly ground black pepper to taste
1 cup apple cider

1. Remove fat from pork. Butterfly pork by cutting in half lengthwise and opening like a book. Do not cut all the way though. Cut in half crosswise to make 2 pieces.
2. Sprinkle with rosemary.
3. Heat oil in a nonstick skillet just big enough to snugly fit the pork. Brown pork on both sides, about 5 minutes total. Salt and pepper the cooked sides.
4. Add cider to the skillet and bring to a simmer. Cover pan with a lid and cook on low for 10 minutes.
5. Remove pork to a plate and raise heat to high. Reduce liquid by half, then spoon sauce over pork.

Exchanges
4 Lean Meat
1 Fruit

Calories	305
Calories from Fat	99
Total Fat	11 g
Saturated Fat	3 g
Cholesterol	97 mg
Sodium	75 mg
Carbohydrate	15 g
Dietary Fiber	1 g
Sugars	13 g
Protein	35 g

Autumn Squash

Preparation time: **25 minutes**
Serves 2/Serving size: **1/2 recipe**

2 tsp olive oil
1 cup fresh or frozen chopped onion
2 cups cubed acorn squash (1/2 inch cubes)
1 Tbsp broken walnuts
Salt and freshly ground black pepper to taste

1. Heat oil in a medium saucepan over medium-high heat.
2. Sauté onions and squash for 8 minutes, stirring several times.
3. Add walnuts and sauté 2 more minutes. Add salt and pepper.
4. Cover and remove from heat. Let sit, covered, for at least 10 minutes or until ready to serve.

Exchanges
1 1/2 Starch
1 Vegetable
1 Fat

Calories	182
Calories from Fat	65
Total Fat	7 g
Saturated Fat	1 g
Cholesterol	0 mg
Sodium	9 mg
Carbohydrate	30 g
Dietary Fiber	9 g
Sugars	12 g
Protein	3 g

PORK

Apricot Fool

Preparation time: **5 minutes**
Serves 2/Serving size: **1/2 recipe**

1/4 cup low-sugar apricot spread
1 cup fat-free artificially sweetened apricot-flavored yogurt
Sugar substitute to the equivalent of 2 tsp

1. Whisk apricot spread in a small bowl.
2. Add yogurt and sugar substitute and whisk until blended. Spoon into small dessert bowls.

Exchanges
1 Carbohydrate
1/2 Fat-Free Milk

Calories 120
  Calories from Fat . . . 0
Total Fat. . . . . 0 g
  Saturated Fat. . . . . . 0 g
Cholesterol. . . . . 2 mg
Sodium. . . . . 87 mg
Carbohydrate. . . . . 25 g
  Dietary Fiber . . . . . . 0 g
  Sugars. . . . . 19 g
Protein. . . . . 5 g

SHOPPING LIST

Produce
1 bunch fresh rosemary
  or 1 bottle dried
  rosemary
1 small acorn squash

Dairy
1 small carton fat-free
  artificially sweetened
  apricot-flavored yogurt

Meat
3/4 lb pork tenderloin

Grocery
1 small package walnuts
1 small bottle apple cider
  (8 oz needed)
1 small jar low-sugar
  apricot spread

STAPLES

Onion
Olive oil
Sugar substitute
Salt
Black peppercorns

italian pork

Italian Roast Pork
Herbed Garlic Lentils
Grapefruit with Toasted Pine Nuts **55 g carb**

This Italian Roast Pork is a simple recipe that goes well with the Herbed Garlic Lentils. Try lentils for a change from rice and other grains. They take only 20 minutes to cook and don't need presoaking.

HELPFUL HINTS

▌ Garlic is used in both recipes, so crush it all at once and divide accordingly.
▌ A quick way to peel a grapefruit is to cut off each end down to the fruit. Stand the grapefruit on a cut end and slice the skin off the sides from top to bottom. Turn on its side and cut into six slices.
▌ Do not overcook the pork or it will become dry and tough. Contrary to what we were all taught when we were younger, pork can be slightly pink inside now. A meat thermometer should read 160°F.

COUNTDOWN

▌ Make lentils
▌ Preheat oven
▌ Roast pork
▌ Make dessert

Italian Roast Pork

Preparation time: **25 minutes**
Serves 2/Serving size: **1/2 recipe**

1 medium clove garlic, crushed
1 Tbsp fresh sage, chopped (or 1/2 Tbsp dried)
3/4 lb pork tenderloin
1 tsp olive oil
Salt and freshly ground black pepper

PORK

1. Preheat oven to 400°F. Line a baking tray with foil.
2. Mix garlic and sage together.
3. Remove fat from pork and cut nearly in half lengthwise. Do not cut all the way through. Open the pork like a book. With a sharp knife, make deep incisions in the pork and insert a little of the garlic-sage mixture in each incision.
4. Brush meat with oil and place on baking tray in the oven. Roast for 15 minutes or until a meat thermometer reads 160°F. Sprinkle with salt and pepper.
5. Slice and serve over the lentils.

Exchanges
4 Lean Meat

Calories	227
Calories from Fat	76
Total Fat	8 g
Saturated Fat	3 g
Cholesterol	97 mg
Sodium	71 mg
Carbohydrate	1 g
Dietary Fiber	0 g
Sugars	0 g
Protein	35 g

Herbed Garlic Lentils

Preparation time: **25 minutes**
Serves 2/Serving size: **1/2 recipe**

1/2 cup dried lentils
2 cups fat-free reduced-sodium chicken broth
1 cup onion, sliced
2 medium cloves garlic, crushed
2 tsp cider vinegar
1 Tbsp olive oil
   Salt and freshly ground black pepper to taste
2 medium tomatoes, sliced

1. Place lentils in a strainer and discard any stones that you find. Rinse and drain.
2. Place a medium saucepan over medium-high heat and add chicken broth. Bring to a rolling boil.
3. Pour lentils into the pot slowly so that the water does not stop boiling. Add the onion and garlic. Reduce heat to medium, cover, and simmer 20 minutes. Check after 15 minutes to see if the pan is dry. Add 1/4 cup water if needed. If there is too much liquid, remove lid and boil to evaporate.

Exchanges
2 Starch
1 Very Lean Meat
2 Vegetable
1 Fat

Calories	276
Calories from Fat	71
Total Fat	8 g
Saturated Fat	1 g
Cholesterol	0 mg
Sodium	518 mg
Carbohydrate	39 g
Dietary Fiber	13 g
Sugars	12 g
Protein	16 g

4. Remove from heat and add vinegar, oil, salt, and pepper. Toss well.
5. Place on individual plates with the sliced pork arranged on top and sliced tomatoes on the side.

Grapefruit with Toasted Pine Nuts

Preparation time: **5 minutes**
Serves 2/Serving size: **1/2 recipe**

1 large grapefruit, peeled and sliced
2 Tbsp pine nuts
  Sugar substitute equivalent to 2 tsp sugar

1. Divide grapefruit slices between 2 dessert plates.
2. Toast pine nuts in a toaster oven or in small skillet until slightly golden, about 1 minute.
3. Sprinkle sugar substitute and pine nuts over grapefruit.

Exchanges
1 Fruit
1 Fat

Calories 107
  Calories from Fat . . 48
Total Fat. . . . . 5 g
  Saturated Fat. . . . . . 1 g
Cholesterol. . . . . . . 0 mg
Sodium. . . . . 0 mg
Carbohydrate. . . . . 15 g
  Dietary Fiber . . . . . . 2 g
  Sugars. . . . . 11 g
Protein. . . . . 3 g

SHOPPING LIST

Produce
1 small bunch fresh sage or 1 bottle ground sage
2 medium tomatoes
1 grapefruit

Meat
3/4 lb pork tenderloin

Grocery
1 small package dried lentils
1 small package pine nuts

STAPLES

Fat-free reduced-sodium chicken broth
Onion
Garlic
Cider vinegar
Olive oil
Sugar substitute
Salt
Black peppercorns

PORK

baked shrimp

Baked Shrimp
Roman Spinach and Orzo
Mocha-Cream Iced Soda

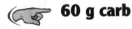 **60 g carb**

This baked shrimp takes less than 15 minutes to make. It is a quick, light dinner using a cooking method that leaves the shrimp juicy, firm, and flavorful.

HELPFUL HINTS

▮ Orzo is small rice-shaped pasta. You can use any type of small pasta or leftover pasta pieces in this recipe.

▮ Buy good quality Parmesan cheese and ask the market to grate it for you or chop it in the food processor. Freeze extra for quick use. You can spoon out what you need and leave the rest frozen.

▮ Buy peeled shrimp from the folks at your seafood counter. If they do not carry peeled shrimp, ask them to peel the shrimp for you. The time saved is worth the slightly higher cost.

▮ Make dessert at the last minute so the soda is fizzy and foamy.

COUNTDOWN

▮ Place water for orzo on to boil
▮ Preheat oven
▮ Boil orzo
▮ Make shrimp
▮ Finish orzo
▮ Make dessert

Baked Shrimp

Preparation time: **15 minutes**
Serves 2/Serving size: **1/2 recipe**

1/2 lb large peeled and deveined shrimp
  2 Tbsp plain bread crumbs
    Salt and freshly ground black pepper to taste
  1 tsp olive oil
1/4 cup dry white wine
  2 Tbsp grated Parmesan cheese

1. Preheat oven to 350°F.
2. Place shrimp in a small baking dish just large enough to hold them in one layer. Sprinkle with breadcrumbs, salt, and pepper. Toss to make sure shrimp is coated with bread crumbs.
3. Drizzle oil over shrimp.
4. Pour wine into baking dish and bake for 10 minutes.
5. Remove from oven and turn on broiler. Sprinkle top with Parmesan cheese and place under broiler for 1 minute. Watch carefully— it will brown quickly!
6. Remove from broiler and serve with orzo and spinach.

Exchanges
1/2 Starch
3 Very Lean Meat
1/2 Fat

Calories 168
  Calories from Fat . . 48
Total Fat. . . . . 5 g
  Saturated Fat. . . . . . 1 g
Cholesterol. . . . . . 179 mg
Sodium. . . . . 302 mg
Carbohydrate. . . . . . 5 g
  Dietary Fiber . . . . . . 0 g
  Sugars. . . . . 1 g
Protein. . . . . 22 g

Roman Spinach and Orzo

Preparation time: **15 minutes**
Serves 2/Serving size: **1/2 recipe**

1/2 cup orzo
10 oz washed ready-to-eat spinach
1/4 cup water
2 Tbsp raisins
2 tsp olive oil
  Salt and freshly ground black pepper to taste

1. Place a medium saucepan 3/4 full of water on to boil for orzo. When water comes to a boil, add orzo and boil 9 to 10 minutes. Drain and set orzo aside.
2. In the same saucepan, place spinach and water and cover. Cook over medium heat 3–4 minutes.
3. Stir in raisins, oil, and orzo.
4. Add salt and pepper and serve.

Exchanges
2 Starch
1 Vegetable
1/2 Fruit
1 Fat

Calories 258
  Calories from Fat . . 51
Total Fat. . . . . 6 g
  Saturated Fat. . . . . . 1 g
Cholesterol. . . . . 0 mg
Sodium. . . . . 114 mg
Carbohydrate. . . . . 43 g
  Dietary Fiber . . . . . . 6 g
  Sugars. . . . . 8 g
Protein. . . . . 10 g

SEAFOOD

Mocha-Cream Iced Soda

Preparation time: **5 minutes**
Serves 2/Serving size: **1/2 recipe**

2 tsp instant decaffeinated coffee
1/2 cup hot water
    Sugar substitute equivalent to 2 tsp
4–5 ice cubes
1/2 cup low-fat chocolate frozen yogurt
8 oz plain soda water (seltzer)

1. Dissolve coffee in hot water.
2. Add sugar substitute and place in refrigerator or freezer to cool for a few minutes.
3. Place ice cubes and coffee mixture in 2 tall glasses.
4. Add frozen yogurt to each glass.
5. Pour soda water over frozen yogurt.
6. Serve with a straw and a long spoon.

Exchanges
1 Carbohydrate

Calories	60
Calories from Fat	7
Total Fat	1 g
Saturated Fat	1 g
Cholesterol	4 mg
Sodium	50 mg
Carbohydrate	12 g
Dietary Fiber	1 g
Sugars	7 g
Protein	2 g

SHOPPING LIST

Produce
1 10-oz package washed ready-to-eat spinach

Seafood
1/2 lb large peeled and deveined shrimp

Grocery
1 small bottle dry white wine
8 oz soda water (seltzer)
1 small package orzo
1 small carton low-fat chocolate frozen yogurt

STAPLES

Parmesan cheese
Plain bread crumbs
Raisins
Decaffeinated instant coffee
Sugar substitute
Olive oil
Salt
Black peppercorns

steamed fish

Chinese Steamed Fish
Spinach and Noodles
Grapefruit with Grand Marnier   **58 g carb**

Juicy, moist, flavorful fish is a Chinese specialty. The Chinese method of steaming helps preserve the fish's delicate flavor and texture. Chinese chefs add flavor with their sauces and vegetables.

This fish is steamed on a dinner plate to hold the juices and sauce. You will need a pot that is wide enough to hold the plate. I find the easiest thing to do at home is place a vegetable steamer opened as flat as possible in a large pot. The plate can then sit on the steamer. Or, you can place the plate on a meat rack in a roasting pan that has a cover.

HELPFUL HINTS

▌ You can use yellowtail snapper or sole instead of flounder in this recipe.

▌ Look for fresh Chinese noodles in the produce department of most supermarkets, or use angel hair pasta instead.

▌ If you prefer, you can use orange juice instead of Grand Marnier or another orange-flavored liqueur for the dessert.

▌ Chopped fresh ginger is used in both recipes, so chop it all at once and divide accordingly.

▌ A quick way to chop ginger is to peel it, cut it into chunks, and press it through a garlic press with large holes. Press ginger over food or a bowl to catch its juices. The ginger pulp will not go through a small garlic press. Just the juice is enough to flavor the dish.

COUNTDOWN

▌ Place water for Chinese noodles on to boil
▌ Make dessert
▌ Steam fish
▌ Make noodles

SEAFOOD

Chinese Steamed Fish

Preparation time: **10 minutes**
Serves 2/Serving size: **1/2 recipe**

3/4 lb flounder fillet
  1 cup thinly sliced button mushrooms
  4 scallions, thinly sliced
  2 tsp chopped fresh ginger
  3 Tbsp dry sherry
  1 tsp lite soy sauce
  1 tsp sesame oil

1. Rinse fish, pat dry, and place on plate that will fit in a steamer.
2. Place vegetables and ginger on top of fish.
3. Mix sherry, soy sauce, and oil together. Pour over fish.
4. Bring water in steamer to a boil, place plate on a steaming rack, and cover.
5. Steam vigorously for 5 minutes.
6. Remove from steamer and serve.

Exchanges
5 Very Lean Meat
1/2 Fruit
1/2 Fat

Calories 217
  Calories from Fat . . 39
Total Fat. . . . . 4 g
  Saturated Fat. . . . . . 0 g
Cholesterol. . . . . . . 89 mg
Sodium. . . . . 249 mg
Carbohydrate. . . . . . 6 g
  Dietary Fiber . . . . . . 1 g
  Sugars. . . . . 3 g
Protein. . . . . 33 g

Spinach and Noodles

Preparation time: **10 minutes**
Serves 2/Serving size: **1/2 recipe**

1/4 lb fresh Chinese egg noodles
  1 tsp sesame oil
  1 tsp chopped fresh ginger
  1 medium clove garlic, crushed
  1 10-oz bag washed ready-to-eat spinach
  2 Tbsp lite soy sauce
     Salt and freshly ground black pepper to taste

1. Bring saucepan half full of water to a boil. Add noodles and simmer 3 minutes or until soft but not sticky. Drain.
2. Heat oil in the same pan and add ginger and garlic. Let cook a few seconds and add spinach.
3. Pour soy sauce over spinach.
4. Add noodles and toss with the spinach, breaking up the spinach leaves with the side of the spoon. Add salt and pepper.
5. Spoon onto plate with fish and serve.

Exchanges
2 Starch
1 Vegetable
1 Fat

Calories 230
   Calories from Fat . . 53
Total Fat. . . . . 6 g
   Saturated Fat. . . . . . 0 g
Cholesterol. . . . . . 54 mg
Sodium. . . . . 831 mg
Carbohydrate. . . . . 37 g
   Dietary Fiber . . . . . . 6 g
   Sugars. . . . . 3 g
Protein. . . . . 13 g

Grapefruit with Grand Marnier

Serve 1/2 large grapefruit sprinkled with 1 Tbsp Grand Marnier (or other orange-flavored liqueur) per person.

SHOPPING LIST

Produce
1 small package
   button mushrooms
   (2 oz needed)
1 bunch scallions
1 small piece fresh
   ginger
1 10-oz bag washed
   ready-to-eat fresh
   spinach
1 large grapefruit
1 package fresh Chinese
   noodles

Seafood
3/4 lb flounder fillet

Grocery
1 small bottle dry sherry
1 small bottle Grand
   Marnier

STAPLES

Garlic
Lite soy sauce
Sesame oil
Salt
Black peppercorns

SEAFOOD

wok shrimp

Wok-Flashed Shrimp
Lemon Basmati Rice
Oranges

 78 g carb

Peppery, stir-fried shrimp served over a bed of tart, lemony rice makes a delicious Chinese dinner. Basmati rice has a fragrant aroma and smells like popcorn when it's cooking. I've added peas to the rice because they're quick and easy to use, but any type of green vegetable will work fine.

HELPFUL HINTS

- You can use any type of white rice.
- Buy peeled shrimp from the folks at your seafood counter. If they do not carry peeled shrimp, ask them to peel the shrimp for you. The time saved is worth the slightly higher cost.
- Chopped fresh ginger is used in both recipes, so chop it all at once and divide accordingly.

COUNTDOWN

- Start rice
- Prepare shrimp ingredients
- Finish rice
- Stir-fry shrimp

Wok-Flashed Shrimp

Preparation time: **10 minutes**
Serves 2/Serving size: **1/2 recipe**

3/4 lb large unshelled shrimp, peeled and deveined
  1 Tbsp cornstarch
1/2 tsp salt
1/4 tsp freshly ground black pepper
  1 Tbsp diced fresh ginger (or 1 tsp ground ginger)
  1 Tbsp canola oil
  5 cloves garlic, crushed

1. Place shrimp in a bowl of water to soak while you prepare the other ingredients. Mix cornstarch, salt, black pepper, and ginger together in a medium bowl.
2. Remove shrimp from water, pat dry with a paper towel, and add to the cornstarch mixture. Toss well to make sure all of the shrimp are covered with the mixture.
3. Heat oil in a wok or skillet on high heat. When oil is smoking, add shrimp and garlic. Stir-fry 4–5 minutes.
4. Serve shrimp over rice.

Exchanges
1/2 Carbohydrate
4 Very Lean Meat
1 Fat

Calories 230
  Calories from Fat . . 82
Total Fat. . . . . 9 g
  Saturated Fat. . . . . . 0 g
Cholesterol. . . . . . 201 mg
Sodium. . . . . 781 mg
Carbohydrate. . . . . 9 g
  Dietary Fiber . . . . . 1 g
  Sugars. . . . . 3 g
Protein. . . . . 27 g

Lemon Basmati Rice

Preparation time: **20 minutes**
Serves 2/Serving size: **1/2 recipe**

1 Tbsp canola oil
1/2 cup basmati rice
2 Tbsp fresh lemon juice
1/4-inch piece fresh ginger
1 cup fat-free reduced-sodium chicken broth
1 cup frozen peas
Salt and freshly ground black pepper to taste

1. Heat oil in a small nonstick skillet over medium heat. Add rice and stir 1 minute.
2. Add lemon juice, ginger, and chicken broth. Bring to a boil, cover, and simmer 10 minutes. Add peas, cover, and cook 5 minutes.
3. Remove ginger, add salt and pepper, and serve.

Exchanges
3 1/2 Starch
1 Fat

Calories 313
Calories from Fat . . 65
Total Fat. . . . . 7 g
Saturated Fat. . . . . . 0 g
Cholesterol. . . . . 0 mg
Sodium. . . . . 323 mg
Carbohydrate. . . . . 54 g
Dietary Fiber . . . . . . 6 g
Sugars. . . . . 5 g
Protein. . . . . 9 g

Oranges

Serve 1 small orange per person.

SHOPPING LIST

Produce
1 small piece fresh ginger
1 lemon
2 small oranges

Seafood
3/4 lb large shrimp

Grocery
1 package basmati rice
1 package frozen tiny
    peas

STAPLES

Garlic
Cornstarch
Canola oil
Fat-free reduced-sodium
    chicken broth
Salt
Black peppercorns

fish soup

Italian Fish Soup (Zuppa di Pesce)
Romaine and Bean Salad
Ginger Apples and Bananas   **79 g carb**

Italian Fish Soup (Zuppa di Pesce) is a perfect soup to warm your insides. Every coastal town in Italy has its own fish soup based on the type of fish found in that area. This aromatic soup is a meal in itself.

For this soup, one type of fish along with some shellfish works best. Of course, the fresher the fish, the better. I have chosen grouper because it is a firm fish that cooks well and is readily available, but you can use any type of non-oily fish that will hold its shape when cooked.

HELPFUL HINTS

▮ You can use any type of beans.
▮ The dessert is made in a microwave oven, which takes only 2 minutes. Or you can bake it in a conventional oven at 400°F for 10 minutes.

COUNTDOWN

▮ Start fish soup
▮ Make salad
▮ Make dessert
▮ Finish soup

Italian Fish Soup (Zuppa di Pesce)

Preparation time: **20 minutes**
Serves 2/Serving size: **1/2 recipe**

2   tsp olive oil
1 cup onion, sliced
1 celery stalk, sliced (about 1/2 cup)
1 carrot, sliced (about 1/2 cup)
1 clove garlic, crushed
1 anchovy fillet
     Several parsley sprigs (about 1/4 cup)
1 cup dry white wine
1 cup clam juice
1/2 lb plum tomatoes, chopped (about 1 1/2 cups)

SEAFOOD

1/2 lb clams (yields 1/4 lb clam meat)
1/2 lb grouper, cut into 3-inch pieces
   Salt and freshly ground black pepper
   2 slices country-style whole grain bread
   Hot pepper sauce to taste

1. Heat oil in a large saucepan over medium-high heat. Add onion, celery, carrot, garlic, anchovy, and parsley. Gently sauté ingredients until onion turns a golden color, about 5 minutes. Do not let the vegetables burn.
2. Carefully stir in wine, clam juice, and tomatoes. Simmer gently for 5 minutes to reduce the liquid.
3. Scrub clam shells. Add clams in their shells and fish. Season with salt and pepper.
4. Bring soup to a simmer, then lower heat and cook, gently, for 5 minutes. Check seasoning and add more, if necessary. Serve in large soup bowls with hot pepper sauce.

Exchanges
1 Starch
5 Very Lean Meat
3 Vegetable
1 Fat

Calories	409
Calories from Fat	81
Total Fat	9 g
Saturated Fat	1 g
Cholesterol	85 mg
Sodium	663 mg
Carbohydrate	33 g
Dietary Fiber	6 g
Sugars	14 g
Protein	43 g

Romaine and Bean Salad

Preparation time: **5 minutes**
Serves 2/Serving size: **1/2 recipe**

1/2 10-oz bag washed ready-to-eat romaine lettuce
1/2 cup cannellini beans, rinsed and drained
   2 Tbsp Paul Newman's Oil and Vinegar Salad Dressing

Combine ingredients in a salad bowl and toss.

Exchanges
1 Starch
1 1/2 Fat

Calories	143
Calories from Fat	75
Total Fat	8 g
Saturated Fat	1 g
Cholesterol	0 mg
Sodium	125 mg
Carbohydrate	12 g
Dietary Fiber	3 g
Sugars	2 g
Protein	5 g

Ginger Apples and Bananas

Preparation time: **5 minutes**
Serves 2/Serving size: **1/2 recipe**

1 small apple, cored and cut into 1/2-inch cubes (1 cup)
1 medium banana, cut into 1/2-inch slices (3/4 cup)
2 tsp butter
4 gingersnaps, crumbled or broken into small pieces
   (2 Tbsp)
2 ramekins or small oven-proof bowls about
   3 × 1 3/4 inches deep

1. Divide apple and banana equally between
   2 bowls.
2. Break butter into small pieces and sprinkle
   on top of fruit.
3. Sprinkle gingersnap crumbs on top.
4. Microwave each bowl separately on high
   1 minute.

Exchanges
1/2 Carbohydrate
1 1/2 Fruit
1 Fat

Calories 181
  Calories from Fat . . 51
Total Fat. . . . . 6 g
  Saturated Fat. . . . . . 2 g
Cholesterol. . . . . . . 10 mg
Sodium. . . . . 131 mg
Carbohydrate. . . . . 34 g
  Dietary Fiber . . . . . . 3 g
  Sugars. . . . . 20 g
Protein. . . . . 1 g

SHOPPING LIST

Produce
1 package carrots
1 package celery
1 small bunch parsley
1/2 lb plum tomatoes
1 small apple
1 medium banana
1 10-oz bag washed
   ready-to-eat Romaine
   lettuce

Seafood
1/2 lb grouper
1/2 lb clams

Grocery
1 tin anchovy fillets
1 small bottle dry white
   wine
1 bottle clam juice
1 box gingersnaps
1 small loaf country-
   style bread
1 can cannellini beans

STAPLES

Onion
Garlic
Butter
Olive oil
Paul Newman's Oil
   and Vinegar Salad
   Dressing
Hot pepper sauce
Salt
Black peppercorns

SEAFOOD

claudine's tilapia

Claudine's Tilapia
Saffron Broccoli and Potatoes
Kiwis with Raspberry Sauce

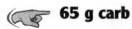 **65 g carb**

Steamed broccoli and potatoes are delicious with the addition of saffron. This side dish is the perfect accompaniment to a sautéed fish fillet with scallion topping. Recently I was visiting the home of television chef Jacques Pepin in Connecticut when their daughter Claudine called to ask how to add a little extra flavor to broccoli. Jacques's wife Gloria told her to steam it and toss it with oil infused with a little saffron. I think you'll agree: the result is delicious!

HELPFUL HINTS

▌ You can use turmeric instead of saffron. The flavor will be different, but still delicious.
▌ Tilapia, also known as St. Peter's fish, is now being farm raised and is available in many supermarkets. It is a flaky white fish. You can substitute any type of non-oily fish in this recipe, such as snapper, sole, or flounder.
▌ You can use frozen raspberries for the dessert, but look for ones frozen without sugar syrup.
▌ If you don't have a steamer, make your own with a large saucepan and a colander. Place the potatoes and broccoli in a metal colander just large enough to sit on the top of the pan with the bottom above the water level.

COUNTDOWN

▌ Start vegetables
▌ Make dessert
▌ Sauté fish
▌ Finish vegetables

Claudine's Tilapia

Preparation time: **10 minutes**
Serves 2/Serving size: **1/2 recipe**

3/4 lb tilapia or other white fish fillet
2 tsp olive oil
  Salt and freshly ground black pepper to taste
2 scallions, sliced
1 lemon, cut into 4 wedges

1. Rinse fish and pat dry with a paper towel.
2. Heat oil in a nonstick skillet over medium-high heat. Add tilapia and sauté 3 minutes. Turn and sauté 3 minutes. Salt and pepper the cooked side.
3. Sprinkle with scallions, cover, and cook 1 minute.
4. Remove tilapia to two dinner plates and squeeze juice from 2 lemon wedges on top. Serve remaining lemon wedge on each plate.

Exchanges
5 Very Lean Meat
1 Fat

Calories 205
  Calories from Fat . . 58
Total Fat. . . . . 6 g
  Saturated Fat. . . . . . 1 g
Cholesterol. . . . . . 89 mg
Sodium. . . . . 148 mg
Carbohydrate. . . . . . 3 g
  Dietary Fiber . . . . . . 1 g
  Sugars. . . . . 1 g
Protein. . . . . 32 g

Saffron Broccoli and Potatoes

Preparation time: **15 minutes**
Serves 2/Serving size: **1/2 recipe**

3/4 lb yellow potatoes
3/4 lb broccoli florets
1 Tbsp olive oil
1/8 tsp saffron threads (8–10 threads)
  Salt and freshly ground black pepper to taste
1/2 cup hot water from steamer

1. Wash potatoes, do not peel, and cut into 1-inch pieces. Place in steaming basket with broccoli. Add 2 inches of water to the base of the steamer or saucepan and add the steaming basket. Cover pot and bring water to a boil. Steam 10 minutes.

(Continued)

Exchanges
2 Starch
2 Vegetable
1 Fat

Calories 249
  Calories from Fat . . 69
Total Fat. . . . . 8 g
  Saturated Fat. . . . . . 1 g
Cholesterol. . . . . . . 0 mg
Sodium. . . . . 52 mg
Carbohydrate. . . . . 41 g
  Dietary Fiber . . . . . . 8 g
  Sugars. . . . . 6 g
Protein. . . . . 8 g

SEAFOOD

2. Heat oil and saffron in a mixing bowl for 15 seconds in a microwave oven, or place bowl over steamer to warm oil and saffron. Add salt and pepper.
3. When potatoes and broccoli are ready, add 1/2 cup steaming water to the oil in the bowl. Add potatoes and broccoli and toss well.

Kiwis with Raspberry Sauce

Preparation time: **5 minutes**
Serves 2/Serving size: **1/2 recipe**

2 kiwi fruit
1 cup fresh raspberries
Sugar substitute equivalent to 1 tsp sugar

1. Purée raspberries in a food processor, food mill, or through a sieve.
2. Add sugar substitute to the purée and spoon onto 2 dessert plates.
3. Peel and slice kiwis and arrange slices on top of purée.

Exchanges
1 1/2 Fruit

Calories 87
  Calories from Fat . . . 7
Total Fat. . . . . 1 g
  Saturated Fat. . . . . . 0 g
Cholesterol. . . . . 0 mg
Sodium. . . . . 5 mg
Carbohydrate. . . . . 21 g
  Dietary Fiber . . . . . . 7 g
  Sugars. . . . . 13 g
Protein. . . . . 1 g

SHOPPING LIST

Produce
1/2 lb yellow potatoes
3/4 lb broccoli florets
1 lemon
1 bunch scallions
2 kiwi fruits
1 small container
  raspberries

Seafood
3/4 lb Tilapia fillets (or
  other white fish fillet)

Grocery
1 small package saffron
  threads

STAPLES

Olive oil
Salt
Black peppercorns

thai snapper

Crisp Thai Snapper
Island Salad
Plum-Glazed Figs

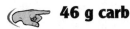 **46 g carb**

Fresh, sweet fish topped with a layer of mustard and golden, crisp, shredded potatoes was one of the dishes I tasted on the Caribbean island of Anguilla, one of the Eastern Caribbean's Leeward Islands. The fishermen go out in their homebuilt boats every day and bring their fresh catches to restaurants and islanders. A simple Thai sauce adds an Asian flavor to the dish.

HELPFUL HINTS

▌ You can use any type of white fish.
▌ Use the grating blade of the food processor or a grater with large holes to shred the potato.

COUNTDOWN

▌ Make dessert
▌ Make snapper dressing
▌ Make salad
▌ Cook snapper

Crisp Thai Snapper

Preparation time: **15 minutes**
Serves 2/Serving size: **1/2 recipe**

1 Tbsp lemon juice
  Sugar substitute equivalent to 1 tsp sugar
2 Tbsp lite soy sauce
1 tsp chopped ginger or 1/2 tsp dried
3/4 lb yellowtail snapper or other light fish fillet, skin removed
2 Tbsp Dijon mustard
1/2 cup shredded russet or Idaho potato (1/4 lb needed)
2 tsp olive oil
  Salt and freshly ground black pepper to taste

(Continued)

Exchanges
1 Starch
5 Very Lean Meat
1/2 Fat

Calories 280
  Calories from Fat . . 67
Total Fat. . . . . 7 g
  Saturated Fat. . . . . . 1 g
Cholesterol. . . . . . . 61 mg
Sodium. . . . . 1046 mg
Carbohydrate. . . . . 14 g
  Dietary Fiber . . . . . . 1 g
  Sugars. . . . . 4 g
Protein. . . . . 38 g

1. In a small bowl, mix lemon juice, sugar substitute, soy sauce, and ginger together and set aside.
2. Rinse fish and pat dry with a paper towel. Spread mustard over one side of fish and place shredded potato on top. Pat potato down so that it is firmly in place.
3. Heat oil over medium-high heat in a nonstick skillet just large enough to hold the fish in one layer. Add fish, potato side up. Sauté 3 minutes. Gently turn fish over and cook 5 minutes to brown potatoes. Salt and pepper the cooked side. Lower heat if potatoes are browning too quickly.
4. Remove fish to individual dinner plates with potato side up. Salt and pepper the potato side. Add sauce from small bowl to the skillet. Warm sauce about 30 seconds and pour over fish.

Island Salad

Preparation time: **5 minutes**
Serves 2/Serving size: **1/2 recipe**

1/2 head Boston lettuce
  1 cup canned hearts of palm, drained and sliced
  2 Tbsp Paul Newman's Oil and Vinegar Salad Dressing

1. Wash and dry lettuce and tear into bite-sized pieces. Place in salad bowl.
2. Add hearts of palm and dressing. Toss and serve with the fish.

Exchanges
1 Vegetable
2 Fat

Calories 113
  Calories from Fat . . 79
Total Fat. . . . . 9 g
  Saturated Fat. . . . . . 1 g
Cholesterol. . . . . . . 0 mg
Sodium. . . . . 480 mg
Carbohydrate. . . . . 7 g
  Dietary Fiber . . . . . 4 g
  Sugars. . . . . 3 g
Protein. . . . . 3 g

Plum-Glazed Figs

Preparation time: **2 minutes**
Serves 2/Serving size: **1/2 recipe**

4 ripe fresh figs
2 Tbsp low-sugar plum spreadable fruit

1. Cut figs into quarters and divide between 2 small dessert plates.
2. Warm spread in a microwave oven on high for 10 seconds or in a saucepan for 30 seconds.
3. Spoon warm spread over fig quarters.

Exchanges
1 1/2 Fruit

Calories 99
  Calories from Fat . . . 3
Total Fat . . . . 0 g
  Saturated Fat . . . . . . 0 g
Cholesterol . . . . 0 mg
Sodium . . . . 12 mg
Carbohydrate . . . . . 25 g
  Dietary Fiber . . . . . . 3 g
  Sugars . . . . 12 g
Protein . . . . 1 g

SHOPPING LIST

Produce
1 lemon
1 small piece fresh ginger or 1 jar ground ginger
1/4 lb russet or Idaho potato
1 head Boston lettuce
4 small figs

Seafood
3/4 lb yellowtail snapper or other light fish fillet

Grocery
1 can hearts of palm
1 small jar low-sugar plum spreadable fruit

STAPLES

Lite soy sauce
Dijon mustard
Sugar substitute
Olive oil
Paul Newman's Oil and Vinegar Salad Dressing
Salt
Black peppercorns

SEAFOOD

seafood kabobs

Seafood Kabobs
Brown Rice
Pear Custard

 64 g carb

Kabobs with a mixture of seafood and colorful vegetables make
a quick, flavorful dinner. I chose shrimp and scallops for their
texture and flavor. Zucchini and yellow squash add color and
crispness. These kabobs need only 5 minutes to cook. The pieces
will be crisp outside and moist and tender inside.

HELPFUL HINTS

- You can use any type of seafood chunks.
- Leave about 1/4 inch between the ingredients on the skewer to allow for even cooking.
- Make sure the grill is hot before cooking the kabobs, or use a hot broiler.
- I like to boil rice like pasta in a pot large enough to let the grains roll freely in the boiling water. This method yields fluffy rice every time.
- To save washing extra bowls, measure milk for dessert in a liquid measuring container and mix remaining ingredients in the same container.

COUNTDOWN

- Preheat oven
- Make rice
- Make dessert
- Marinate kabobs
- Preheat grill
- Grill kabobs

Seafood Kabobs

Preparation time: **25 minutes**
Serves 2/Serving size: **1/2 recipe**

- **2** Tbsp lime juice
- **1** Tbsp olive oil
- **1** clove garlic, crushed
- **1/8** tsp salt
- **1/4** tsp freshly ground black pepper

2 tsp fresh snipped dill
12 large shelled deveined shrimp (6 oz meat)
7 large sea scallops (6 oz)
1 medium zucchini cut into 1-inch pieces (2 cups)
1 medium yellow squash cut into 1-inch pieces (2 cups)

1. Preheat grill or broiler.
2. Mix lime juice, olive oil, garlic, salt, pepper, and dill together.
3. Add shrimp, scallops, and vegetables and set aside to marinate for 15 minutes. Turn once during this time.
4. Alternate vegetables, shrimp, and scallops on 4 skewers. Grill or broil 3–4 inches from the heat source for 2 1/2 minutes per side. Do not overcook the fish. Sprinkle with salt and pepper.
5. Place skewers on 2 dinner plates or remove seafood and vegetables from skewers onto 2 plates and serve.

Exchanges
4 Very Lean Meat
2 Vegetable
1/2 Fat

Calories 224
 Calories from Fat . . 42
Total Fat . . . . 5 g
 Saturated Fat . . . . . . 0 g
Cholesterol . . . . . . 157 mg
Sodium . . . . 314 mg
Carbohydrate . . . . . 12 g
 Dietary Fiber . . . . . . 4 g
 Sugars . . . . 7 g
Protein . . . . 34 g

Brown Rice

Preparation time: **35 minutes**
Serves 2/Serving size: **1/2 recipe**

1/2 cup quick-cooking 30-minute brown rice
2 tsp olive oil
 Salt and freshly ground black pepper to taste

1. Fill a medium saucepan halfway with cold water and add rice. Bring water to a boil and gently boil rice for about 30 minutes. Test a few grains to see if they are cooked through but still firm.
2. Drain, leaving a little water on the rice. With a fork, stir in oil, salt, and pepper.

Exchanges
2 1/2 Starch
1/2 Fat

Calories 210
 Calories from Fat . . 54
Total Fat . . . . 6 g
 Saturated Fat . . . . . . 1 g
Cholesterol . . . . 0 mg
Sodium . . . . 3 mg
Carbohydrate . . . . . 35 g
 Dietary Fiber . . . . . . 2 g
 Sugars . . . . 0 g
Protein . . . . 5 g

SEAFOOD

Pear Custard

Preparation time: **35 minutes**
Serves 2/Serving size: **1/2 recipe**

1 ripe pear, peeled, cored, and cut into 1-inch pieces
(1 cup)
1/2 cup fat-free milk
Sugar substitute equivalent to 1/2 tsp sugar
1/2 tsp vanilla extract
1 egg
1 Tbsp walnut pieces

1. Preheat oven to 350°F.
2. Place pear pieces in 2 ramekins or small oven-proof bowls about 3 × 1 3/4 inches deep. Mix fat-free milk, sugar substitute, vanilla extract, and egg together and pour on top of pears.
3. Sprinkle walnuts on top and bake 30 minutes or until custard is firm.
4. Remove from oven, allow to cool a few minutes, and serve.

Exchanges
1 Carbohydrate
1 Fat

Calories 135
  Calories from Fat . . 47
Total Fat . . . . 5 g
  Saturated Fat . . . . . . 1 g
Cholesterol . . . . . . 108 mg
Sodium . . . . 64 mg
Carbohydrate . . . . . 17 g
  Dietary Fiber . . . . . . 2 g
  Sugars . . . . 13 g
Protein . . . . 6 g

SHOPPING LIST

Produce
1 lime
1 medium zucchini
1 bunch fresh dill
1 medium yellow squash
1 ripe pear

Seafood
6 oz large shelled shrimp
6 oz large sea scallops

Grocery
1 small package walnut
  pieces

STAPLES

Garlic
Fat-free milk
Eggs
Olive oil
Sugar substitute
Vanilla extract
Quick-cooking 30-minute
  brown rice
Salt
Black peppercorns

scallops

Sautéed Scallops
Saffron Vegetable Pilaf
Mocha Froth

 65 g carb

Sweet, tender scallops need very little cooking. In fact, to remain delicate and flavorful, they should be cooked only a few minutes over high heat in a skillet large enough to hold them in one layer without touching. This results in scallops with a crusty coating and juicy insides.

HELPFUL HINTS

▌ You can substitute turmeric for saffron. Although the pilaf flavor will be different, the dish is still very good.
▌ You can use small bay scallops instead of large sea scallops, but reduce cooking time to 1 minute per side.

COUNTDOWN

▌ Start pilaf
▌ Make scallops
▌ Finish pilaf
▌ Make dessert just before serving

SAUTÉED SCALLOPS

Preparation time: **10 minutes**
Serves 2/Serving size: **1/2 recipe**

2 tsp olive oil
3/4 lb large scallops
1/2 Tbsp flour
1/2 cup dry vermouth
1/2 cup fat-free reduced-sodium chicken broth
2 Tbsp heavy cream
Salt and freshly ground black pepper to taste

1. Heat oil in a nonstick skillet over medium-high heat. Add scallops and sauté 2 1/2 minutes on each side.

(Continued)

Exchanges
1/2 Carbohydrate
4 Very Lean Meat
2 1/2 Fat

Calories 300
 Calories from Fat . 101
Total Fat. . . . . 11 g
 Saturated Fat. . . . . . 4 g
Cholesterol. . . . . . 77 mg
Sodium. . . . . 406 mg
Carbohydrate. . . . . . 8 g
 Dietary Fiber . . . . . . 0 g
 Sugars. . . . . 6 g
Protein. . . . . 29 g

2. Remove scallops to a plate and add flour to pan.
3. Add vermouth to the pan, raise heat to high, and reduce liquid by half, about 1 minute. Add chicken broth and reduce by half again, about 1 minute. Remove from heat and stir in cream. Add salt and pepper.
4. Return scallops to the pan just to warm through, about 1/2 minute, and serve.

Saffron Vegetable Pilaf

Preparation time: **20 minutes**
Serves 2/Serving size: **1/2 recipe**

   1 tsp olive oil
1/2 cup fresh or frozen chopped onion
1/2 cup portobello mushrooms, sliced
1/2 cup long-grain white rice
   1 cup fat-free reduced-sodium chicken broth
1/4 tsp saffron threads
   1 cup frozen peas
       Salt and freshly ground black pepper to taste
   2 Tbsp freshly grated Parmesan cheese

1. Heat oil in a nonstick skillet over medium-high heat. Add onion and mushrooms. Sauté 3 minutes.
2. Add rice and sauté 1 minute.
3. Add chicken broth and saffron.
4. Bring liquid to a simmer, cover, and cook 10 minutes. Add peas and continue to simmer, covered, for 3 minutes. Liquid should be absorbed and rice cooked through. Simmer a few more minutes if needed.
5. Add salt and pepper, sprinkle with Parmesan cheese, and serve with scallops.

Exchanges
3 Starch
1 Vegetable
1/2 Fat

Calories 303
  Calories from Fat . . 42
Total Fat. . . . . 5 g
  Saturated Fat. . . . . . 1 g
Cholesterol. . . . . 5 mg
Sodium. . . . . 369 mg
Carbohydrate. . . . . 53 g
  Dietary Fiber . . . . . . 6 g
  Sugars. . . . . 8 g
Protein. . . . . 12 g

Mocha Froth

Preparation time: **5 minutes**
Serves 2/Serving size: **1/2 recipe**

1 cup boiling water
2 tsp instant decaffeinated coffee
   Sugar substitute equivalent to 2 tsp sugar
1/2 cup fat-free milk
10 ice cubes

1. Pour water into a blender and add coffee and sugar substitute.
2. Blend several seconds, then add the milk and ice cubes. Blend until thick, about 1 minute.
3. Pour into tall glasses and serve with a straw and long spoon.

Exchanges
Free Food

Calories	26
Calories from Fat	1
Total Fat	0 g
Saturated Fat	0 g
Cholesterol	1 mg
Sodium	32 mg
Carbohydrate	4 g
Dietary Fiber	0 g
Sugars	3 g
Protein	2 g

SHOPPING LIST

Produce
1 small package portobello mushrooms

Dairy
1 small carton heavy cream

Seafood
3/4 lb large scallops

Grocery
1 small package saffron threads
1 small bottle dry vermouth
1 package frozen peas
1 package frozen chopped onion

STAPLES

Parmesan cheese
Fat-free milk
Olive oil
Flour
Long-grain white rice
Decaffeinated instant coffee
Sugar substitute
Fat-free reduced-sodium chicken broth
Salt
Black peppercorns

SEAFOOD

shrimp creole

Shrimp Creole
Brown Rice
Carambola Cooler

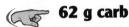 **62 g carb**

Fresh shrimp in a spicy tomato sauce is a classic New Orleans dish. Carambola Cooler, a refreshing tropical drink, provides a satisfying conclusion to the meal.

HELPFUL HINTS

- Buy peeled shrimp from the folks at your seafood counter. If they do not carry peeled shrimp, ask them to peel the shrimp for you. The time saved is worth the slightly higher cost.
- Buy tomato paste in a tube. You can use a small amount and store the rest of the tube in the refrigerator until you need it again.
- You can use any hot pepper sauce, in any quantity you can stand!
- Carambolas are also called star fruit. They are usually available from August to mid-February. Use strawberries as a substitute.

COUNTDOWN

- Purée carambola and refrigerate
- Make rice
- Make shrimp
- Assemble dessert

Shrimp Creole

Preparation time: **20 minutes**
Serves 2/Serving size: **1/2 recipe**

- **1** Tbsp canola oil
- **1** cup onion, sliced
- **1** cup green pepper, sliced
- **2** medium cloves garlic, crushed
- **2** cups diced tomatoes
- **1/2** Tbsp tomato paste
- **2** Tbsp water

1/2 Tbsp Worcestershire sauce
1 tsp hot pepper sauce
3/4 lb medium peeled and deveined shrimp

1. Heat oil in medium nonstick skillet over medium-high heat. Add onion, green pepper, and garlic and sauté 3 minutes.
2. Add tomatoes and sauté another 5 minutes.
3. Mix tomato paste with water and add to skillet along with Worcestershire and hot pepper sauce. Cook 1 minute.
4. Add shrimp and sauté 2–3 minutes.
5. To serve, spoon shrimp and sauce over rice.

Exchanges
4 Very Lean Meat
3 Vegetable
1 1/2 Fat

Calories 277
  Calories from Fat . . 81
Total Fat. . . . . 9 g
  Saturated Fat. . . . . . 0 g
Cholesterol. . . . . . 261 mg
Sodium. . . . . 385 mg
Carbohydrate. . . . . 19 g
  Dietary Fiber . . . . . . 4 g
  Sugars. . . . . 11 g
Protein. . . . . 31 g

Brown Rice

Preparation time: **35 minutes**
Serves 2/Serving size: **1/2 recipe**

1/2 cup quick-cooking 30-minute brown rice
2 tsp canola oil
  Salt and freshly ground black pepper to taste

1. Fill a large saucepan 3/4 full of water, bring to a boil, and add rice.
2. Gently boil rice for about 30 minutes or according to package instructions. Test a few grains to see if they are cooked through, but still firm.
3. Strain into a colander, leaving a little water on the rice.
4. Add oil, salt, and pepper.

Exchanges
2 1/2 Starch
1/2 Fat

Calories 210
  Calories from Fat . . 54
Total Fat. . . . . 6 g
  Saturated Fat. . . . . . 1 g
Cholesterol. . . . . . . 0 mg
Sodium. . . . . 3 mg
Carbohydrate. . . . . 35 g
  Dietary Fiber . . . . . . 2 g
  Sugars. . . . . 0 g
Protein. . . . . 5 g

SEAFOOD

Carambola Cooler

Preparation time: **5 minutes**
Serves 2/Serving size: **1/2 recipe**

1/2 lb ripe carambolas (2 medium or 5 small; 2 cups chunks yield
    1/2 cup juice)
  2 tsp sugar substitute
1/2 cup soda water (seltzer)
  4 ice cubes

1. Wash carambola and slice 2 stars from the center of the largest fruit. Set aside for garnish.
2. Cut remaining fruit into large chunks. Place in food processor with sugar substitute and process 2 minutes or until fruit is turned into a pulpy juice. Strain into glass, being sure to press as much juice as possible from the pulp. Place in refrigerator until needed or up to 8 hours.
3. When ready, add soda water and ice cubes to the glasses.
4. Cut a slit halfway through each reserved star and stick it on the side of the glass as a garnish. Serve immediately.

Exchanges
1/2 Fruit

Calories 36
   Calories from Fat . . . 3
Total Fat. . . . . 0 g
   Saturated Fat. . . . . . 0 g
Cholesterol. . . . . 0 mg
Sodium. . . . . 14 mg
Carbohydrate. . . . . . 8 g
   Dietary Fiber . . . . . . 3 g
   Sugars. . . . . 6 g
Protein. . . . . 1 g

SHOPPING LIST

Produce
1 medium green pepper
2 medium tomatoes
1/2 lb carambolas
   (2 medium or 5 small)

Seafood
3/4 lb medium peeled and
   deveined shrimp

Grocery
1 can or tube tomato
   paste
1 small bottle soda water
   (seltzer)

STAPLES

Onion
Garlic
Quick-cooking 30-minute
   brown rice
Canola oil
Worcestershire sauce
Hot pepper sauce
Sugar substitute
Salt
Black peppercorns

mahi-mahi

Herb-Crusted Mahi-Mahi
Vegetable Brown Rice
Apricot-Glazed Pears

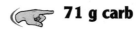 **71 g carb**

When fish is really fresh, it needs only a few minutes to cook. Add fresh herbs and you have a quick, delicious meal.

HELPFUL HINTS

- You can use any type of non-oily fish fillet in this recipe. Count 10 minutes cooking time for each inch of thickness. To check for doneness, stick the point of a knife into the flesh. If the flesh is opaque, it is ready.
- You can use green beans, zucchini, or any other green vegetable instead of broccoli.
- The dessert is best with any type of ripe pear, but it can be made with semi-ripe ones. Add sugar substitute equivalent to 1 tsp to the lemon juice if pears are not fully ripe.

COUNTDOWN

- Make rice
- Preheat broiler
- Broil fish
- Make dessert

Herb-Crusted Mahi-Mahi

Preparation time: **15 minutes**
Serves 2/Serving size: **1/2 recipe**

	Olive oil cooking spray
3/4	lb mahi-mahi fillets
2	tsp olive oil
2	Tbsp pine nuts
1/4	cup chopped fresh parsley
	Salt and freshly ground black pepper to taste

1. Preheat broiler.
2. Line a baking sheet with foil and spray it with cooking spray. Place mahi-mahi on sheet and spray it with cooking spray.
3. Place sheet under broiler about 3–4 inches from heat source. Broil 5 minutes on each side for a piece 1 inch thick.
4. Heat oil in a small skillet on medium heat and add pine nuts. Sauté 1 minute or until pine nuts start to turn golden. Remove from heat and toss with parsley.
5. Remove mahi-mahi and divide between 2 dinner plates. Add salt and pepper. Spoon pine nuts and herbs on top.

Exchanges
5 Very Lean Meat
1 1/2 Fat

Calories 247
  Calories from Fat . . 98
Total Fat. . . . . 11 g
  Saturated Fat. . . . . . 2 g
Cholesterol. . . . . . 131 mg
Sodium. . . . . 162 mg
Carbohydrate. . . . . . 2 g
  Dietary Fiber . . . . . . 1 g
  Sugars. . . . . 0 g
Protein. . . . . 36 g

Vegetable Brown Rice

Preparation time: **35 minutes**
Serves 2/Serving size: **1/2 recipe**

1 1/2 cups water
1/2 cup quick-cooking 30-minute brown rice
1/2 lb broccoli florets
  Salt and freshly ground black pepper to taste
1/2 cup fat-free plain yogurt

1. Place water in a medium saucepan over high heat. Add rice and bring to a boil.
2. Reduce heat to medium and cover. Simmer 25 minutes.
3. Add broccoli and continue to cook, covered, 5 minutes. All of the water should be absorbed and the rice cooked through.
4. Add salt, pepper, and yogurt. Toss well.

Exchanges
2 1/2 Starch

Calories 212
  Calories from Fat . . 14
Total Fat. . . . . 2 g
  Saturated Fat. . . . . . 0 g
Cholesterol. . . . . 1 mg
Sodium. . . . . 62 mg
Carbohydrate. . . . . 41 g
  Dietary Fiber . . . . . . 2 g
  Sugars. . . . . 5 g
Protein. . . . . 9 g

Apricot-Glazed Pears

Preparation time: **10 minutes**
Serves 2/Serving size: **1/2 recipe**

2 ripe pears
1 tsp butter
2 Tbsp lemon juice
2 Tbsp low-sugar apricot spread

1. Core and slice pears.
2. Heat butter in a medium nonstick skillet over medium heat and add the pear slices. Sauté 1 minute.
3. Mix lemon juice with apricot spread and add to skillet. Toss to coat pears.
4. Cover skillet and cook 5 minutes or until pears are soft. Divide between 2 dinner plates and pour juice on top.

Exchanges
2 Fruit
1/2 Fat

Calories	 128
Calories from Fat	. . 22
Total Fat	. . . . 2 g
Saturated Fat	. . . . . . 1 g
Cholesterol	. . . . 5 mg
Sodium	. . . . 34 mg
Carbohydrate	. . . . . 28 g
Dietary Fiber	. . . . . . 3 g
Sugars	. . . . 22 g
Protein	. . . . 1 g

SHOPPING LIST

Produce
1 bunch parsley
1/2 lb broccoli florets
2 ripe pears
1 lemon

Dairy
1 carton fat-free plain yogurt

Seafood
3/4 lb mahi-mahi fillets

Grocery
1 small package pine nuts
1 small jar low-sugar apricot spread

STAPLES

Olive oil cooking spray
Olive oil
Butter
Quick-cooking 30-minute brown rice
Salt
Black peppercorns

SEAFOOD

key west shrimp

Key West Shrimp
Quick Coleslaw
Strawberries and Cream
  Angel Food Cake   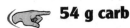 **54 g carb**

Succulent, fresh pink shrimp are a trademark of the Florida
Keys. This is a never-fail recipe for tasty shrimp.

It's a breeze to fix homemade coleslaw if you use shredded,
ready-to-eat cabbage and carrots from the supermarket, but
I prefer to add my own dressing. Store-bought coleslaw is usually dripping with mayonnaise and sometimes has added sugar.

HELPFUL HINTS

▌ You can use any type of shrimp.
▌ If you don't have Key lime juice, just use
  regular lime or lemon juice.

COUNTDOWN

▌ Make coleslaw
▌ Boil shrimp
▌ Make sauce
▌ Make dessert

Key West Shrimp

Preparation time: **10 minutes**
Serves 2/Serving size: **1/2 recipe**

  6 Tbsp ketchup
    Several drops hot pepper sauce
  1 Tbsp plus 2 tsp Key lime juice, divided
3/4 lb large peeled and deveined shrimp

1. Mix ketchup, hot pepper sauce, and 2 tsp
   Key lime juice together in a small bowl.
2. Fill a medium saucepan 3/4 full with water.
   Add shrimp and 1 Tbsp Key lime juice. Make
   sure water covers shrimp. Add more water if
   needed.

Exchanges
1 Carbohydrate
4 Very Lean Meat

Calories 182
  Calories from Fat . . 16
Total Fat . . . . 2 g
  Saturated Fat . . . . . . 0 g
Cholesterol . . . . . . 261 mg
Sodium . . . . 834 mg
Carbohydrate . . . . . 13 g
  Dietary Fiber . . . . . . 1 g
  Sugars . . . . 5 g
Protein . . . . 29 g

3. Bring water to a simmer with bubbles just starting around the edge of the pot (the water will start to turn white). Remove pot from heat immediately and let sit 1 minute.
4. Drain shrimp and plunge into cold water if serving cold, or serve immediately if serving hot. Serve with sauce.

Quick Coleslaw

Preparation time: **5 minutes**
Serves 2/Serving size: **1/2 recipe**

2 Tbsp mayonnaise
1/4 cup white vinegar
1 Tbsp Dijon mustard
Sugar substitute equivalent to 1 tsp sugar
Salt and freshly ground black pepper to taste
2 cups shredded ready-to-eat cabbage
1/2 cup shredded ready-to-eat carrots
1/2 cup red onion, sliced

1. Mix mayonnaise, vinegar, mustard, sugar substitute, salt, and pepper together in a medium bowl.
2. Add cabbage, carrot, and onion and toss well. Taste for seasoning and add more if necessary.

Exchanges
2 Vegetable
2 1/2 Fat

Calories 156
  Calories from Fat . 106
Total Fat. . . . . 12 g
  Saturated Fat. . . . . . 1 g
Cholesterol. . . . . 9 mg
Sodium. . . . . 283 mg
Carbohydrate. . . . . 13 g
  Dietary Fiber . . . . . . 3 g
  Sugars. . . . . 8 g
Protein. . . . . 3 g

Strawberries and Cream Angel Food Cake

Preparation time: **5 minutes**
Serves 2/Serving size: **1/2 recipe**

1 2 × 2 × 3-inch piece angel food cake (1 1/2 oz), sliced
in half
1 cup sliced strawberries
Sugar substitute equivalent to 2 tsp sugar
2 Tbsp whipping cream

1. Place cake slices on 2 plates.
2. Mix strawberries, sugar substitute, and cream
together and spoon over cake.

Exchanges
2 Carbohydrate
1 Fat

Calories 174
  Calories from Fat . . 54
Total Fat. . . . . 6 g
  Saturated Fat. . . . . . 3 g
Cholesterol. . . . . . . 21 mg
Sodium. . . . . 73 mg
Carbohydrate. . . . . 28 g
  Dietary Fiber . . . . . . 2 g
  Sugars. . . . . 17 g
Protein. . . . . 4 g

SHOPPING LIST

Produce
1 red onion
1 bag washed shredded
  ready-to-eat cabbage
1 bag shredded ready-to-
  eat carrots
1 small package fresh
  strawberries

Dairy
1 small carton whipping
  cream

Seafood
3/4 lb large peeled and
  deveined shrimp

Grocery
1 bottle Key lime juice
1 small angel food cake

STAPLES

Mayonnaise
Dijon mustard
Ketchup
Hot pepper sauce
Sugar substitute
White vinegar
Salt
Black peppercorns

index
alphabetical list of recipes

Linguine, 104
Litchi Cup, 95

M

Marinated Mushroom Salad, 101
Mediterranean Egg Salad Sandwich, 68
Mediterranean Meat Loaf, 105
Microwave Ham-Scrambled Eggs, 4
Middle Eastern Meatballs, 115
Mocha Froth, 167
Mocha Slush, 107
Mocha-Cream Iced Soda, 146
Mojo Roasted Pork, 135

N

Neapolitan Pizza, 76
Norwegian Bagel Breakfast, 26
Nutty Cinnamon French Toast, 30

O

Oatmeal, 3

P

Parmesan Frittata, 6
Parmesan Tomatoes and Beans, 131
Pasta and Bean Soup (Pasta e Fagioli), 88
Peach Skewers, 119
Pear Custard, 164
Pears with Pineapple Sauce, 137
Picadillo, 126
Plum-Glazed Figs, 161

Q

Quick Coleslaw, 175
Quick Stir-Fried Rice, 122
Quick Turkey Wrap, 64

R

Roast Beef Sandwich with Tomato and Corn
    Relish, 74
Romaine and Bean Salad, 154
Roman Spinach and Orzo, 145

S

Saffron Broccoli and Potatoes, 157
Saffron Vegetable Pilaf, 166

Salsa Beef Salad, 52
Sausage and Tortellini Soup, 84
Sautéed Scallops, 165
Seafood Kabobs, 162
Shrimp and Black-Eyed Pea Salad, 36
Shrimp Caesar Salad, 42
Shrimp Creole, 168
Shrimp Roll, 62
Smoked Fish Salad, 44
Smoked Salmon Omelet, 18
Smoked Turkey Waldorf Salad, 46
Southwestern Chicken, 96
Spiced Berries, 98
Spicy Grilled Cheese and Tomato Sandwich, 22
Spinach and Mushroom Omelet, 16
Spinach and Noodles, 148
Steak and Portobello Mushroom Sandwich, 70
Strawberries and Cream Angel Food Cake, 176
Strawberry-Banana Cup, 131
Stuffed Veal Rolls, 130
Sweet Tequila Sunrise, 113
Swiss Omelet, 12

T

Tangy Chicken and Pear Salad, 56
Toasted Almond Chicken Salad, 50
Toasted Turkey Breakfast Sandwich, 28
Tomato and Onion Salad, 127
Tomato, Onion, and Basil Frittata, 10
Tomato-Cheese Melt, 25
Tortilla Salad, 97
Turkey and Goat Cheese Enchiladas, 78
Turkey and Vegetable Soup with Cheddar
    Bruschetta, 86
Turkey Chili, 112
Tuscan Bean and Tuna Salad with Tomatoes,
    38

V

Veal Gorgonzola, 133
Vegetable Brown Rice, 172

W

Warm Zucchini Salad, 116
Wok-Flashed Shrimp, 151

subject index

About the American Diabetes Association

The American Diabetes Association is the nation's leading voluntary health organization supporting diabetes research, information, and advocacy. Its mission is to prevent and cure diabetes and to improve the lives of all people affected by diabetes. The American Diabetes Association is the leading publisher of comprehensive diabetes information. Its huge library of practical and authoritative books for people with diabetes covers every aspect of self-care—cooking and nutrition, fitness, weight control, medications, complications, emotional issues, and general self-care.

To order American Diabetes Association books: Call 1-800-232-6733. Or log on to http://store.diabetes.org

To join the American Diabetes Association: Call 1-800-806-7801. www.diabetes.org/membership

For more information about diabetes or ADA programs and services: Call 1-800-342-2383. E-mail: Customerservice@diabetes.org or log on to www.diabetes.org

To locate an ADA/NCQA Recognized Provider of quality diabetes care in your area: www.ncqa.org/dprp/

To find an ADA Recognized Education Program in your area: Call 1-888-232-0822. www.diabetes.org/recognition/education.asp

To join the fight to increase funding for diabetes research, end discrimination, and improve insurance coverage: Call 1-800-342-2383. www.diabetes.org/advocacy

To find out how you can get involved with the programs in your community: Call 1-800-342-2383. See below for program Web addresses.

- *American Diabetes Month:* Educational activities aimed at those diagnosed with diabetes—month of November. www.diabetes.org/ADM
- *American Diabetes Alert:* Annual public awareness campaign to find the undiagnosed—held the fourth Tuesday in March. www.diabetes.org/alert
- *The Diabetes Assistance & Resources Program (DAR):* diabetes awareness program targeted to the Latino community. www.diabetes.org/DAR
- *African American Program:* diabetes awareness program targeted to the African American community. www.diabetes.org/africanamerican
- *Awakening the Spirit: Pathways to Diabetes Prevention & Control:* diabetes awareness program targeted to the Native American community. www.diabetes.org/awakening

To find out about an important research project regarding type 2 diabetes: www.diabetes.org/ada/research.asp

To obtain information on making a planned gift or charitable bequest: Call 1-888-700-7029. www.diabetes.org/ada/plan.asp

To make a donation or memorial contribution: Call 1-800-342-2383. www.diabetes.org/ada/cont.asp